If Only I Had Known

Integrative & Alternative
Paths to Recovery
from **Breast Cancer**

AVIVA MAYERS, M.S.W.
Foreword by Alvin Pettle, M.D.

◆ FriesenPress

Suite 300 - 990 Fort St
Victoria, BC, V8V 3K2
Canada

www.friesenpress.com

Foreword by Alvin Pettle, M.D.

ISBN
978-1-5255-4676-1 (Hardcover)
978-1-5255-4677-8 (Paperback)
978-1-5255-4678-5 (eBook)

1. *Medical, Oncology, Breast Cancer*

Distributed to the trade by The Ingram Book Company

DEDICATION

To my friends Nina, Marjolein, Gerry, and all the women who have died too young of breast cancer. If only they had known...

And to my beloved dog Sweet Pea, a calming presence, always at my side, keeping a watchful eye as I wrote and re-wrote, and who himself as I was finally completing this book, succumbed to cancer.

TESTIMONIALS

This wonderful book explores conventional treatment as well as alternative therapy. The research is excellent. I would like to see this book in waiting rooms for breast surgeons, oncologists, radiologists and radiation therapists. It would provide much comfort and information to patients dealing with the many facets of breast cancer and its treatment.

—Patricia H. Saluk, MD, Mammography/Radiology, Southeast Radiology Ltd., Upland, PA, USA

As someone who has undergone breast cancer treatment using conventional and alternative methods myself, it is so refreshing to finally read something that validates the importance of integrative and alternative treatments—with expert opinions and substantive research to back it up. I wish I'd had this book when I was first diagnosed as it would have saved me much anxiety around choosing the best treatment path for my body and my disease.

—Rosalind Stefanac, patient, journalist

TABLE OF CONTENTS

When diagnosed with breast cancer, I found myself travelling the well-worn conventional path of treatment, only to spend years subsequently undoing the ravages of those treatments with alternative interventions.

In contrast to my story, Lori opted for carefully timed surgery and an alternative path thereafter. She refused chemotherapy, radiation, and adjuvant hormonal therapy and remained well with no recurrence at the time of completing her interview for this book, more than nine years after her initial diagnosis.

> **Adjuvant therapy**
> Adjuvant therapy is administered after surgery to decrease the risk of recurrence or metastasis. Examples include chemotherapy, radiation, and hormonal interventions.

Bernard sought help from the Chinese doctor and herbalist Dr. Ma Hong Chau in Hong Kong following an unsuccessful conventional treatment for stage IV colon cancer that had spread to his liver. After a year-long treatment with Dr. Ma, he was pronounced cured, and remains well at the time of completing this book 13 years after his initial diagnosis.

A world-renowned naturopath in the treatment of breast cancer, Sat Dharam Kaur pays meticulous attention to diet and supplementation. She employs various blood and urine tests to monitor health status and to prevent recurrences and metastases.

Dr. Pettle is a pioneer in Canada in the use of bio-identical hormones, their utility in the prevention of breast cancer, and its recurrence after the initial onset. He believes that managing disorders of the hormonal system such as elevated cortisol and depleted DHEA are crucial in preventing cancer.

Bio-identical hormones, which are made from a chemical extracted from yams and soy, have an identical molecular structure to hormones that are naturally produced by the body.

Dr. Mostovoy, who trained at the Homeopathic College of Canada, pioneered the use of thermograms in Canada. Thermograms are a safe screening tool and early warning system for breast cancer. In his work, he addresses the individual on a psycho-emotional, biophysical, and biochemical level to enable the body to self-correct.

Dr. Nasri, homeopath, naturopath and trained in medicine and surgery, is the founder of the Nasri Integrative Medicine Clinic located in Woodbridge, in greater Toronto. He employs a holistic approach to treating patients that considers their history, genetics, environment, and lifestyle. Dr. Nasri discusses how he integrates alternative treatments into mainstream oncology with his cancer patients.

Dr. Hui's practice is influenced by his early years spent in Hong Kong, as well as his subsequent medical training and practice in Canada. He discusses some of the innovative complementary and alternative practices that he discovered in different parts of the globe that contribute to the well-being, and in some instances, the recovery of patients with cancer.

> Complementary medicine includes those non-mainstream health care practices and substances that may be used alongside mainstream medical treatments. When alternative practices are combined with mainstream medicine they are considered complementary. Alternative practices are those treatments or substances that are used instead of mainstream medicine practices. Alternative therapies are generally considered less likely to harm the body than certain conventional therapies. Alternative therapies can include treatments such as homeopathy, osteopathy, acupuncture, reiki, aromatherapy, naturopathy and others.

Dr. Charles Hayter, a radiation oncologist and a medical historian, encourages the medical community to give patients a voice and choice in their treatment. He stresses the importance of this by bringing to light the story of oncologist Vera Peters. Peters' research, first published in mid-1970's and revolutionary for that time, showed that lumpectomy could be as safe for some patients as mastectomy in the treatment of breast cancer.

Chapter 10: Dr. Shailendra Verma, Medical Oncologist

A medical oncologist at the Ottawa Hospital Cancer Centre, Dr. Verma underscores that the time is right for both conventional and complementary health care professionals to collaborate on research and clinical interventions with patients.

Chapter 11: Biological Dentistry

Dental materials and procedures in the mouth and oral bacteria can affect health throughout the body. In this chapter, several biological dentists offer their views on safe, science-based treatments and dental materials that contribute to good health.

FOREWORD

Alvin Pettle, MD

The mainstream medical model for treating breast cancer is outdated and is overly influenced by the background clatter of machinery and drug choices of the day. The main tools employed by medical doctors in the treatment of breast cancer are surgery and drugs. Hospitals are replete with machinery that is over-utilized because an army of people is employed for its operation and hospitals rely on the income such machinery generates. While tools such as mammograms have their place in making a diagnosis, each time you irradiate a woman's breast, you are pushing her closer to the very thing you are trying to prevent: a cancer diagnosis. The indiscriminate use of, for example, birth control pills in young women or hormone replacement therapy in menopausal women, has also contributed to giving cancer to our mothers and daughters. As medical doctors, I believe we have been complicit in this abuse and, therefore, in its adverse consequences.

The call of the future requires medical doctors to have the courage to look beyond the medical system currently in place. Medical schools teach doctors to view disease as something that has to be removed, rather than a condition that can be predicted and, therefore prevented by really getting to know the patient. When faced with a patient with cancer, surgery and drugs are the doctor's treatments of choice. If the first drug doesn't work, the patient is given a second drug, and maybe a third, in an effort to save his or her life. But cancer doesn't occur overnight. What doctors observe must be seen in the context of the whole of the patient's life. The transition from normal physiology to pathology and cancer is a process that begins at least ten to fifteen years earlier, when the immune system is depressed. Each patient brings a unique story to the table, and doctors must get to know the person who has the disease — history, genetics, diet, and lifestyle — putting aside old protocols and preconceived ideas on how to treat this disease.

This is a book about courageous professionals who are treating patients with breast cancer with integrative and alternative methods and are experiencing amazing successes. This book illuminates the work of those practitioners who, like Dr. Frederick Banting and Dr. Charles Best, have dared to work with cancer in unique ways and in doing so are changing medical history.

The practitioners interviewed offer a variety of important interventions that may contribute to both the prevention and treatment of breast cancer, as well as other cancers. Unfortunately, when a patient is diagnosed, too often he or she must contend with a regimented health care system that conveys the message: "If you don't do what I say, you will die." No medical doctor has the capacity to adequately process the myriad of information available regarding the diagnosis and treatment of breast cancer. Making such pronouncements can prevent some patients from following a path to recovery that intuitively makes sense for them, which many believe could be an important psychological ingredient in healing. This book brings us steps closer to helping patients unravel the mass of information out there. If you are a patient, it will help you to choose a course of treatment for your illness that resonates with you. It will inform you of options outside of conventional medicine; options that you will see can be very effective in halting or reversing cancer without the collateral damage that conventional treatments inflict.

This book will take you to a future health care system that we would like to see, where there will be an openness on the part of the medical establishment to other ways of intervening in the disease. Here, the patient will be at the centre of a wheel of treatment, the radiating spokes inhabited by medical doctors working with naturopaths, homeopaths, acupuncturists, and many others. A multiplicity of professionals from all ends of the spectrum will contribute to a treatment plan that makes sense, both intellectually and intuitively, to the patient.

I would like to give my heartfelt thanks to all health care providers who continue to dedicate their lives to helping families through any and all cancers.

Dr. Alvin Pettle

PREFACE

Approximately 26,000 women in Canada are diagnosed annually with breast cancer and almost a quarter of those die from it. More women develop breast cancer than any other form of cancer, except for certain skin cancers, and younger women are increasingly stricken with this disease.

> Younger women are defined in the breast cancer literature as below 35 or 40 years[1]

A diagnosis is overwhelming, and those who receive it find themselves hurtling down a well-travelled system, facing choices about radical, debilitating treatment. They are given little time to adequately apprise themselves of the real benefits or pitfalls of treatment or to educate themselves about alternative interventions that may be less invasive and less toxic. Cancer takes years to show itself (10 – 15 is the standard amount that is cited), and for many cancers, there is time after diagnosis to become informed about treatment options and choose a course of action that makes sense to you. This can have psychological benefits that may ultimately contribute to a better outcome. Many consider patients cured if they remain cancer-free for the first five years after their initial diagnosis. The reality, however, is that cancer can recur in any individual at any time and be lethal. Oncologist Siddhartha Mukherjee, notes in an article in The New Yorker Magazine that when

---

1   Gabriel, C. A., & Domchek, S. (2010). Breast cancer in young women. *Breast Cancer Research, 12*(5), 212. https://doi.org/10.1186/bcr2647.

surgeons remove a breast tumour, and there is no sign of a spread of the cancer to the lymph nodes in the armpits, a patient will be classified by the oncologist as N.E.D, that is "no evidence of disease".[2] But this classification may be misleading, as it refers rather to our understanding at this point in time about the disease, rather than the actual state of the disease. Cancer cells that may not show up on scans or tests, could have escaped and spread to other organs. Women who fall under this classification of N.E.D can have a metastasis at any point in the near or distant future. He also points out that because doctors are unable to predict whether a cancer will become metastatic, too many patients are treated with toxic chemotherapy as if it is a certainty that they will have a metastasis when only a fraction might benefit. Given this lack of certainty, it seems crucial that sufferers be informed of the full range of treatment possibilities.

Siddhartha Mukherjee is an oncologist and author of the Pulitzer Prize-winning book *The Emporer of All Maladies: A Biography of Cancer*

This book explores integrative and alternative medical treatment options available to women who have been diagnosed with breast cancer as well as to their caretakers and loved ones. It is also a guide to finding practitioners and treatments that you, the reader, may not hear about from medical doctors. It will help fully inform women who have been recently diagnosed and must make a quick decision about a course of treatment, as well as women at all other stages of the disease. Those who have completed a conventional course of treatment and wish to consider health-restoring interventions will also find this book helpful. With the information contained in these pages, women may gain an increased sense of control over a truly frightening experience. A heightened sense of control helps to generate hope,

2   Mukherjee, S. (2017, September 11). Cancer's Invasion Equation. *The New Yorker*. Retrieved from https://www.newyorker.com/magazine/2017/09/11/cancers-invasion-equation

an important psychological ingredient in outcome. The treatment options discussed in this book do not represent an exhaustive list, but offer a taste of the many options that are available mostly in Canada, but also in other places around the world. As breast cancer diagnoses reach near epidemic proportions around the world, it is crucial that we be apprised of, and examine carefully all options available for its treatment, management and prevention. This will contribute to healing on both a psychological, and physical level in all those who are struggling with this disease.

> Integrative medicine is the combination of conventional and alternative therapies. It also considers the whole person, that is mind, body and lifestyle.

The writing of this book emerged out of my own experience following a conventional course of treatment for a diagnosis of breast cancer eleven years prior to the completion of this book. As the uncertainty and fear regarding my own diagnosis receded, the seeds for this book took root. I have spent many years since my diagnosis undoing the ravages of the treatment with integrative and alternative treatment regimes. Throughout this time I have explored and reflected at great length on missed opportunities due to my confusion, fear, and lack of information at the time of diagnosis. I am now convinced that, had I been better informed early in my diagnosis about all treatment possibilities, I would have made different choices.

As my understanding of the many facets of breast cancer and its treatments grew, so has my wish to prevent other women from unnecessarily undergoing debilitating treatments such as those that I endured, which represent the current "standard of care" in mainstream medicine. As I witness other women receiving repeated bouts of chemo and radiation for their breast cancer and becoming increasingly debilitated in direct relation to the rounds of treatment, I wonder how the immune system can possibly recover from such a toxic barrage. While I believe there is a place for these interventions, they are highly toxic, and it is well known that they inflict much collateral damage, sometimes contributing to an early death. This places their usefulness in question. I believe it is time that mainstream medicine adopt a more critical stance towards its standard protocols for this disease. This stance should explore and include, as warranted, the work of integrative and alternative practitioners who have had success in treating breast cancer and other cancers. There is currently little research on the usefulness of more natural, less invasive, and less costly alternatives to conventional treatment. Additionally, there is not enough encouragement from many mainstream doctors to explore these avenues, either as an adjunct to or in lieu of the conventional route. As long as the successes of integrative and alternative practitioners are ignored, some "standard of care" treatments will remain inadequate. In the meantime, women must be made aware of a range of treatment options in a timely fashion, given the radical and debilitating nature of many conventional therapies.

"Standard of care" or "standard care" treatment is the package of treatments that are routinely suggested for most breast cancers and includes some combination of surgery, radiation, chemotherapy and hormone suppressing medication. The particular package may vary from one institution to another

This book includes interviews with professionals who treat women with breast cancer using both integrative and alternative medicine. Many of those interviewed are leading practitioners in their fields in Canada. I personally conducted the interviews, taking handwritten notes and simultaneous tape recordings in order to accurately obtain the verbatim account provided by the interviewee. While the interviews are mostly verbatim, in some cases I synthesized what the professionals said for further clarity. After transcribing the interviews, I checked their accuracy where possible with the practitioners.

In these interviews, they discuss their views on the interventions employed in conventional medicine, the services they offer to breast cancer patients, their thoughts on combining multiple medical interventions, and their advice to newly diagnosed women. I also interviewed medical doctors in the field of conventional oncology who are receptive to certain integrative and alternative treatments.

The chapter on biological dentistry is important because oral health is crucial in overall health. Biological dentists believe that toxic materials used in dental procedures such as root canals can have a profound effect on overall health and may contribute to the genesis of illness elsewhere in the body, including breast cancer.

The section in this book entitled "The Well Worn Path" presents data regarding certain breast cancer prevention and treatment options that doctors often do not discuss with patients. The data presented here conflict with some of the standard protocols used by doctors during treatment, casting uncertainty on some of these choices, which might lead patients to make different choices if fully informed.

I hope that you, the reader, will find this book to be a useful guidepost in thinking about and seeking treatment for breast cancer in a fundamentally different way.

Part I

A Breast Cancer Diagnosis:
Two Journeys

CHAPTER 1

My Story

My experience at the time of diagnosis mirrors that of the majority of other newly diagnosed women. I visited the hospital for my annual appointment in the familial breast cancer study. Since my mother had breast cancer in her sixties, I was flagged as high-risk, though it was never something I worried about too much. On this particular occasion, the breast surgeon who was examining me as I lay on the consulting room table awoke me from my reverie.

"I feel a thickening," she said, motioning to the medical student to feel also, but she reassured me that she thought it was likely nothing.

Shortly after, I was sent for an ultrasound. There, the chief radiologist who was called in for a second opinion announced that she couldn't find anything worrisome on the ultrasound. Given the family history, she suggested they do a further procedure to be sure. Soon I was shuffled off for a core biopsy, and as I lay on the gurney, a doctor twisted a needle deep in my chest. The procedure was painful and tears rolled down my cheeks, fear enveloping me as I read consternation in her face. But when the procedure was finished, I got dressed and left the hospital, reminding myself I was a healthy person, trying to leave any worries about my health behind as I re-joined the busy world outside.

I still remember clearly the phone call that jolted me from my busy workday two weeks after the needle biopsy. It was the doctor calling me from her cottage. Perhaps taking this unusual measure to inform me outside of her normal work hours was an indication of how surprised she was by the results. Her solemn voice caused my heart to skip a beat.

"I didn't expect this," she said, "but it's cancer."

I broke down sobbing. Me and cancer. I was still reeling from the recent dissolution of my marriage, and the breast cancer diagnosis hit me like an aftershock. From that moment on, I was caught in a whirlwind of hospital appointments, second opinions, and surgery. I was encouraged to follow the customary route of chemotherapy, radiation, and hormone therapy.

> Hormone therapy is used with a breast cancer that is hormone receptor positive. This means that the breast cancer cells are positive for either estrogen or progesterone or both. The hormone therapy can prevent hormones from attaching to breast cancer cells and can also decrease the body's production of hormones.[3] In my case, tamoxifen was recommended..

As the survival statistics were thrown at me in the midst of this crisis, I looked to authoritative voices to guide me. The loudest voices came from the medical establishment — oncologists, surgeons, and general medical doctors. Despite the uncertainty attached to some of the suggestions made by these professionals, I felt inclined to follow their suggestions due to my fear.

The business-like oncologist I was referred to ventured no opinion on which chemotherapy might be most suitable for me, and gave me scant indication of the debilitating side effects of the treatment. Finally she left the consulting room when I burst into tears contemplating the road ahead. In my confusion, I agreed to six rounds of chemotherapy, only to downgrade it to four before I began. I felt I was in a race, as my friends found women who had also been through breast

---

3   Hormonal therapy for breast cancer. *Canadian Cancer Society.*
      Retrieved from http://www.cancer.ca/en/cancer-information/
      cancer-type/breast/treatment/hormonal-therapy/?region=on

cancer treatments and sent them to talk to me and cheer me on to the finish line. The evening after my first round of chemotherapy I began vomiting uncontrollably. I ended up in the emergency room and was told I had been overdosed with the chemotherapy by about 20%. In retrospect this miscalculation may have occurred because the weight I had been losing due to fear and anxiety had not been considered, thereby resulting in an incorrect dosage. When I emerged from the fog and terror related to the diagnosis and treatment, I was well on my way down the conventional path. The chemotherapy was more debilitating than I could have imagined, and doubts about what I had agreed to grew as the treatment proceeded.

Chemotherapy

Chemotherapies, many of which are derived from poisonous mustard gas, are very toxic agents that act by interfering with cell division in order to bring about cell death (apoptosis). The effects of mustard gas on soldiers was initially reported on during World War I, however pharmacologists became interested in its use as a cancer treatment during World War Two. This followed the discovery that people exposed to this gas during a bombing campaign in Southern Italy suffered decimated white blood cells and depleted bone marrow.

In the course of my treatment, a radiologist friend suggested I pick up the book *Anticancer: A New Way of Life* by David Servan-Schreiber. The author's moving story and the questions he raised about conventional medicine opened up a new world to me and filled me with hope. Suddenly I realized there were other ways to manage this frightening disease. Rather than bombarding the immune system with toxins, and in so doing killing healthy cells as well as malignant ones, I learned that it is possible to adopt a gentler, more holistic approach that bolsters an ailing immune system. This made sense to me.

Throughout my treatment, I attended healing classes at Wellspring, a privately funded cancer support organization that has branches in both Ontario and Alberta. It is an oasis of calm amid the sea of uncertainty that a new cancer diagnosis brings. As my contacts in the integrative and alternative world grew, I eventually found my way to Sat Dharam Kaur, a naturopathic doctor who has written an internationally recognized, well-documented, and extensive work on preventing and treating breast cancer using the naturopathic model. I came into contact with women who were following alternative treatments to manage their cancer, and I reflected on my mother's experience. Thirty-two years ago she was diagnosed with her first bout of breast cancer. It had spread to her lymph nodes under her arm and she agreed to have surgery and radiation, refusing chemotherapy. She was placed on tamoxifen, an estrogen suppressing hormonal therapy, which was administered to prevent a recurrence. However, three years later, while still on the tamoxifen, she had a recurrence, so tamoxifen was terminated. She had one more recurrence more than twenty years later in her thyroid, with spread to the nodes. This was also treated with surgery and radiation. She is alive and thriving, age ninety-three, at the completion of this book, and attributes her survival to the daily intake of propolis, a bee product that is a mix of bee saliva, beeswax and resin from the buds of conifer and poplar trees. It is believed to have immune boosting properties. Through all of these women's experiences, I realized that less harsh treatment options worked for some people. The stories of these women are inspiring, yet there is a marked dearth of research both on this population, and the professionals who helped them on their way.

I began to wonder why this useful information is not readily available in hospitals, as a matter of course, in addition to standard procedures and options presented to breast cancer patients. My dismay at this shortcoming led me to ask more and more questions. In doing so, I set out on a path of discovery and empowerment.

This book is the product of my search and serves as a guidepost for women who themselves have a diagnosis of breast cancer or who have friends or relatives with breast cancer. If you are in this situation, it will inform you and offer you a range of options for both before and after treatment. With this information, you can choose what makes sense to you, rather than simply follow the conventional, well-worn path due to fear, lack of information, and what has been called the "burden of choice" one is faced with when refusing what is referred to as the "standard of care" treatment.[4] This book also offers useful tips on how you can prevent getting breast cancer in the first place.

4   Mayne, C. (2009). On being diagnosed with breast cancer. *Breast Cancer Action, winter.* Retrieved from https://bcaction. org/2009/12/21.on-bing-diagnosed-with-breast-cancer

CHAPTER 2

Lori's Story

I found myself travelling a well-worn conventional path of treatment for my breast cancer, only to spend years subsequently undoing damage done by those treatments with alternative interventions. Lori, on the other hand, a nurse from Midland, Ontario, opted for carefully timed surgery and an alternative path thereafter. She refused chemotherapy, radiation, and estrogen suppressing medication and remained well at the time of this interview, nine years after her diagnosis. The following is her story.

Lori was no stranger to the health care field when she received a diagnosis of breast cancer at the age of forty-eight. She had been a nurse for twenty-four years, and during that time, assisted her sister in determining a course of treatment for her diagnosis of breast cancer. Well-armed with much information about the disease, Lori's own diagnosis eleven years after her sister's still came as a shock. "I ate well. I jogged. I had an overconfident feeling it couldn't happen to me," says Lori, who recalled feeling numb when she received the diagnosis. She struggled with what to tell her son, feared she might die, and relived the trauma of her mother's death from colon cancer when Lori was thirteen.

When I spoke with Lori, there was a quiet determination about her that I guessed had served her well in resisting the pressure of conventional medicine in the treatment of her cancer. "I'm not a person to follow the rules," she said. "It probably goes back to my mother's death. I went through a rebellion then. I'm not a sixties child, but I'm part of that movement." Her inquisitive nature had set the stage for her choices later, and she recalls being influenced by John Robbins's book *Diet for a New America*. "It exposed a lot of medical stuff. I read that the famous Sloan-Kettering Cancer Center in New York got huge donations from someone who owned a radium mine in the early nineteen hundreds. I feel we are all being duped."

When Lori was first diagnosed, she took time to assess her treatment options. "When you are newly diagnosed with breast cancer, you're not even thinking; you feel like a deer in the headlights. But you have time to research. Don't panic. You don't need to jump and run." She discovered research suggesting that surgery is more successful when progesterone is high and estrogen is low.[5,6] Her surgeon agreed to consider this when scheduling her surgery. Lori consulted a family member, a surgeon at the Mayo Clinic, who told her that if she followed the Clinic's protocol — that is, radiation and tamoxifen — she'd increase her life by four to six years. "The US is known to be more aggressive, but the Mayo Clinic didn't recommend chemotherapy," says Lori, "and I figured I'd get the same recommendations in Barrie. But instead, they were more aggressive here, recommending chemotherapy and radiation after surgery. If I decided against these recommendations, they suggested a mastectomy.

"I had felt there was a universal standard, but now I realized it's up to the individual oncologist. It was a shocking revelation. I knew people who had done part or all of chemo and had irreparable damage. There is a lot of research that says chemotherapy doesn't do well on solid tumours and survival rates haven't changed in fifty years. It was

---

5   Kucuk, A. L., & Atalay, C. (2012). The relationship between surgery and phase of the menstrual cycle affects survival in breast cancer. *Journal of Breast Cancer, 15*(4), 434-40. https://doi.org/10.4048/jbc.2012.15.4.434

6   Fentiman, I. S. (2002). Timing of surgery for breast cancer. *International Journal of Clinical Practice 56*(3), 188-90.

assembly-line medicine: this is what you take, this is where you get the wig… It left me with a pit in my stomach."

Lori decided against chemotherapy. "I thought I could be wrong and one day that I might go that route, but I didn't want the cure to kill me and I wanted my immune system to remain intact. The oncologists have to offer everyone the "standard of care". Once they've informed the patient of this standard, they are satisfied they've done their job with respect to the liability piece. Some doctors become hostile and indignant when patients don't follow their recommendations, but my doctor was kind and respectful. I didn't have to defend myself or feel diminished in any way."

The conflicting information Lori received concerning her treatment options made her recall her sister's experience of receiving differing advice on treatment options at Johns Hopkins University Hospital in Baltimore and Princess Margaret Hospital in Toronto. "My doctor wanted to put me on tamoxifen, but I wasn't going down that path either," said Lori. "My sister's doctor said tamoxifen was a personal choice, but my doctor said, 'All my breast cancer patients are on tamoxifen.'"

Motivated by fear and desperation, Lori recalls exploring many avenues outside mainstream medicine. Initially she consulted a homeopath, a naturopathic doctor, and an integrative medicine gynecologist. The homeopath helped her reduce trauma and promoted healing after the surgery, while the gynecologist followed her closely with blood work and ultrasound. Then, more conflicting advice presented itself. The gynecologist prescribed bio-identical hormones, including progesterone, but the naturopathic doctor deemed this risky. Feeling overwhelmed by the volume of remedies prescribed for her by the three practitioners she was consulting, Lori allowed herself to be guided mostly by the naturopath, Sat Dharam Kaur.

Homeopathy is a system in which a patient is given very small, curative doses of a substance that in larger doses would be harmful.

Lori drank Essiac tea, the main ingredients of which include sheep sorrel and burdock root. This tea was first used by Canadian nurse Rene Caisse in the 1920s to successfully treat cancer patients at all stages. More recently, the tea was made famous by President John F. Kennedy's personal physician, Dr. Charles Brusch, who claimed in the 1980s that consuming it cured his own cancer. Lori also took resveratrol, a substance that has anti-cancer properties and is found in grapes, berries, and other plant sources; and Wobenzym, a tablet containing plant-based enzymes that some say boosts the immune system. " The idea is that cancer cells hide or wall themselves off from circulating immune cells like NK cells and macrophages", says Lori. "Wobenzym breaks down these walls so that the NK cells will recognize the cancer cells and attack them." Lori was also interested in Iscador, an anti-cancer treatment that is derived from mistletoe and is widely used in Northern Europe for its anti-tumour and immune-boosting properties, but she was unable to pursue that due to the high cost. For the first couple of years, mindful of the stress coffee places on the adrenal glands, she drank green tea instead. This helped move her body from an acid environment where cancer cells thrive, into an alkaline one where cancer cells cannot survive.

The cells of the innate immune system

Basophils and eosinophils
These two types of cells play complementary roles in defending against parasites and reacting to allergens.

Gamma/Delta T cells
Little is known yet about these complex cells, other than that they may bridge the gap between our innate immune system, which defends us from infection in general, and our adaptive immune system, which learns from past infections in preparation for future attacks.

Mast cells
These reside in our mucus membranes and connective tissue. Their primary roles are to heal wounds, fight pathogens, and react to allergens.

Natural killer cells
Ominously named, but here to help, NK cells, a type of white blood cell, ideally kill intruders such as cells infected with viruses or those destined to form tumours.

Phagocytes
Phagocytes, which include macrophages (Greek for "big eater"), neutrophils, and dendritic cells, are scavenger cells that gather at sites of infection and remove bacteria and other foreign bodies.

Throughout Lori's experience with cancer, she read voraciously and was influenced by books such as Theodore Brody's *Alkalize or Die*, John R. Lee's *What Your Doctor May Not Tell You about Breast Cancer: How Hormone Balance Can Help Save Your Life*, Samuel Epstein's *Cancer Gate*, Sandra Steingraber's *Living Downstream*, and Jozef Krop's *Healing the Planet One Patient at a Time*. Dr. Krop notes that dealing with mercury (in amalgam fillings) in the mouth, detoxing, and eating well are all crucial places to start.

Lori cites luck and a rebellious streak for many of her choices. "People showed up in my life at the right time. I had my first mammogram at twenty-three for a lump and had consulted a surgeon who was really ahead of his time and questioned why I was having a mammogram at my age. He said the breast is bio-sensitive, and there was a possibility that radiation from the mammogram could damage the DNA in breast tissue. That struck me, and I don't do mammograms anymore. I do MRIs and annual thermograms."

Prevention and management of breast cancer is like tending a garden, says Lori. "You need the right soil conditions for it to grow. I think diet is huge, and stress. I feel more of an affinity to food as medicine, and mind-body approaches. To protect myself now, I don't drink [alcohol], I try to eat well, I don't eat processed foods, no dairy, and no meat with hormones. Sugar and cancer is a bad combo. I've looked at raw cuisine." She is influenced by Jane Plant's story. Plant, a British scientist and outspoken advocate for altering diet to prevent cancer, herself had more than a half dozen recurrences of cancer over 22 years. She attributed her surviving so many recurrences to altering both her lifestyle and diet, which included dropping dairy from her diet. "But I don't think it's that simple," says Lori, reflecting on the role she believes emotional turmoil played in affecting her recovery from surgery. "No sooner had I got in the door from the breast cancer surgery when I got the phone call to say my dad had passed away from lung cancer. I ended up with a hematoma in my breast."

Though Lori was determined to not follow a conventional course of treatment, other than surgery, she feels humble about the choices she did make. "I've always felt in my heart there are infinite possibilities for healing. Everybody should find their own path. When you refuse conventional treatment, a huge part of healing is feeling you have passion and purpose." In Lori's case, the conventional treatment recommended for her after surgery consisted of chemotherapy, radiation, and hormonal therapy.

"My emotional life is different since the cancer diagnosis. I've looked into Ayurvedic approaches and more spiritual dimensions such as Kundalini yoga, meditation, even chanting. At first I thought chanting was far out; then after the first weekend I realized how powerful it was. I've learned to keep an open mind."

When I interviewed Lori for this book, it had been nine years since she had been diagnosed with cancer. "Initially I had a lot of times when I'd wake up fearful and overwhelmed, but my attitude now is I can face whatever it is. I've dealt with death as a nurse. It doesn't scare me. I struggle with resisting salt and sugar, but I don't stew over it. I feel it's a crapshoot, I could have a recurrence next week, but if I did I would probably do it differently now. I wouldn't have a needle biopsy; I believe that releases cancer cells around the body. Maybe I'd use a cancer salve to draw out the cells. We are our own healers, and the body has an innate ability to heal."

The conventional medical world is often uncertain about the outcomes of breast cancer treatments such as chemotherapy, radiation and mastectomy. Lori's story illustrates how, despite the pressure to adhere to standard of care treatments, a breast cancer sufferer can achieve a good outcome by choosing integrative or alternative options.

CHAPTER 3

Bernard's Story

Bernard, a retired civil servant in Hong Kong, requested help from Dr. Ma Hong Chau, an herbalist and registered traditional Chinese medicine doctor. Bernard sought this help, following an unsuccessful conventional treatment for stage IV colon cancer that had spread to his liver. He felt the hospital had sent him home to die, but he'd always been an optimistic person and wasn't ready to give up. After a year-long treatment with Dr. Ma, Bernard was pronounced cured. When I met him twelve years later, he was well and thriving, cancer free.

I have included Bernard's story in this book about breast cancer because Dr. Ma, the Chinese doctor who treated Bernard, has also successfully treated many other cancers, including breast cancer.

One morning in August, 2005, Bernard went to fetch the morning paper as he always had. He bent down and was suddenly racked with indescribable pain. He was rarely ill, so he passed it off as a transient case of food poisoning and assumed he'd be better in the morning. However, the pain persisted and became more unbearable, so his wife called an ambulance. Bernard was operated on the next day and seeking relief, gave the surgeons free rein. He awoke to the shocking news that he had colon cancer and that part of his colon had been removed during surgery, leaving him with a temporary colostomy. "I seldom went to the doctor because I was rarely sick," says Bernard. "I always considered myself a lucky man." However, the cancer had spread to his liver, and a month later a liver resection was performed.

It was pronounced a success, and ten days later he was discharged with a clean bill of health, allegedly cancer free.

"As a precaution afterward," says Bernard, "I was referred to the oncology department for follow-up, where I was advised to do chemotherapy to ensure all the cancer was completely gone and would not return. I agreed to follow a course of twelve visits, two days each, with a chemotherapy drug that was administered over a forty-eight-hour period". Despite being told that the chemo would eliminate any leftover cancer cells, an abdominal ultrasound conducted after Bernard had completed nine rounds of chemo, revealed that the cancer had returned and that there was another tumour on the liver. This occurred six months after the initial diagnosis, and Bernard was advised to have a third surgery to remove two-thirds of the liver. "This operation was major," says Bernard. "It was my third operation in nine months, and I was in intensive care afterwards, but again I was told after the surgery that the markers were normal and I was clear. Two weeks after the surgery I was discharged, but when I asked the oncologist if I should take the remaining three chemos, he said it was pointless because the cancer had returned during chemo. According to the doctors, this meant that because of the nature of the cancer, the chemo had no positive effect on it. Now I felt that orthodox medicine had reached its limit, and I was just waiting for the cancer to return, for the final call, which would be indicated by another recurrence." It was at this point that Bernard began searching for other solutions. A friend of Bernard knew of Dr. Ma Hong Chau, an herbalist and registered traditional Chinese medicine doctor. He had built a reputation in China and in his clinic in Hong Kong, where he helped people with cancer to go into remission. Bernard decided to consult him.

"Hong Kong is a society that adheres to the Western medicine model for treating illness," said Bernard. "If you get sick, usually you go to a mainstream medical doctor and he prescribes medication. Not many people in Hong Kong would trust traditional Chinese medicine to treat a cancer illness, so people seldom consult it. In fact, not many traditional Chinese doctors are competent to treat a cancer, so conventional doctors don't see traditional Chinese medicine as an option. In Hong Kong, Chinese medicine is considered more of a supplementary treatment, for soothing your discomfort, or to make you healthier and stronger over a long period of time. Dr. Ma believes that the flu virus, if left untreated, can gradually gather force inside the body, and find its way to a particular organ, springing attack, and perhaps spreading to other organs afterwards. There is a diagnosis in Chinese that says that 'the flu got into your inner system,' and the implication of this is that this may give rise to adverse consequences, the worst of which is cancer developing in one or more organs. Dr. Ma believes that if a patient seeks treatment as soon as the common flu symptoms, such as feeling sick, sneezing, coughing, or rising body temperature present themselves, the flu could easily be kept under control and swept away. Treatment at this point might include three to five doses of a particular herbal tea. If the patient delays treatment, that might require seven to fourteen doses of the herbal tea to get healed. In the worst case scenario, if the patient doesn't seek treatment to address the problem at all, the virus may, over time, develop into a cancer. Dr. Ma believes that food poisoning is another symptom of being infected with this virus. Cancer can develop in the body from food poisoning in the same manner as infection with the flu virus. He says the cause of the majority of pancreatic cancers he has treated is food poisoning. He believes that eating inappropriate foods opens the way for infection. Consequently, his treatment draws the toxins out of the system for the body to heal. He feels we need to target the whole body and detox it, not just the localized cancer."

"People come to Dr. Ma by word of mouth, and he sees about one hundred patients daily in his clinic between the hours of four and seven. He charges 100 HK dollars (about $13 US) for a consultation, and herbs cost about 80 HK dollars, but if you have trouble paying, he will waive the charges. It seems the quality of his herbs is very high as he sources, stores, and processes the herbs he uses himself."

"The first thing Dr. Ma did was check my pulse and examine my neck. Then he asked me to get an X-ray of the neck. He believes all cancer patients have a disorder of the neck caused by poor blood flow and misalignment, and this in turn affects the immune system. Based on the X-ray, which Dr. Ma read, I had treatments to restore my neck to its proper position from trained therapists in Dr. Ma's office. At every visit, he read my pulse and determined the herbal prescription. At the end of the treatment, the pulse was restored to normal. According to traditional Chinese medicine, some part of the system is not functioning properly and the internal organs are in disorder. Dr. Ma believes herbs help to rectify the problem by detoxifying the body. Xiao is the basic herb, but he prescribes others to deal with different problems. I had to drink tea comprised of certain herbs. Then after one half-hour Dr. Ma performed acupuncture to facilitate the detox process. There were dietary restrictions while taking the herbs. He advised me against things like lobster, cold foods, and sour foods. For some people, the detoxifying happens through the nervous system, and that can cause pain and discomfort. For instance, they may suffer swollen legs, which in turn can cause difficulty walking, and that can affect their morale. As supplementary treatment, I received acupuncture for about three years to clear out the toxins inside my body."

"Dr. Ma's method isn't guaranteed. I was lucky because the herbal treatment didn't give me any problems. The doctor is trying his best to treat people, but I've seen successes and failures. I have witnessed a patient with pancreatic cancer fully recover in one month after following Dr. Ma's healing process. In another case, a man who sought Dr. Ma's help for the treatment of liver cancer recovered fully after following Dr. Ma's treatment. This included taking an herbal tea for about three years. The hospital which was following this case was astonished that the tumour had disappeared. These patients did not have either chemotherapy or radiation. I have also seen cases where the treatment failed after a year or two."

"My colostomy was removed after I completed the Chinese medicine course, about two years after it was inserted. At the end of 2006, after a year of treatment with Dr. Ma, I was declared cancer free. Between 2006 and now, I've had inspections at the hospital for conventional medicine every six to nine months, including x-rays and four colonoscopies. I got a clean bill of health on each occasion."

"When I had a recurrence at the time I was undergoing treatment after my initial diagnosis, I was told by doctors there was nothing that could be done and I had only a 30 percent chance of survival. Now conventional doctors count me lucky, but I don't tell them I went to an herbal doctor. I attribute my recovery in part to the herbalist's ability to diagnose me correctly and prescribe the right herbs. I entrusted myself to the herbalist, a factor which I think is very important, because you must believe in whatever you do. Initially I entrusted myself to conventional medicine because I didn't know anything about herbal medicine. I was amazed at that time that if there were eight or ten people doing chemo at the same time, they were all having the same chemo drugs. It made me suspicious that the doctors were prescribing the same thing for different people. Sometimes I think doctors are too influenced by drug companies. Nevertheless, I feel it was my destiny to go through these different treatments. I think one important aspect of recovery is to take a relaxed attitude, to remain composed and not worry. Perhaps my recovery was one-half herbs and one-half attitude. I didn't rely solely on medicines or herbs. Taking drugs is not a big deal, and medical treatment is only part of the story, but dealing with cancer is also a mind game. One must stay positive, cheerful, and generally healthy mentally, and that is more difficult. Many patients give up too easily and sink into despair. I exercise to strengthen my body and my mind; it fosters the fighting spirit which we need to deal with the cancer. I do Chi Gong and Tai Chi, and I massage my body with my own hands, in particular, the chi (energy) points. Even during the treatment, I did light exercise. You need to do something yourself to take control."

Part II

Breast Cancer Prevention and Treatment: The Practitioners' Perspectives

CHAPTER 4

Sat Dharam Kaur, Naturopath

Sat Dharam Kaur is an internationally recognized expert in the field of complementary and alternative treatments for breast cancer. She is a graduate of the Canadian College of Naturopathic Medicine, holds both BSc and BA degrees, and has developed a healthy breast program to educate women about naturopathic ways to prevent and treat breast cancer. She teaches, consults, and travels the world in her tireless efforts as an advocate for non-invasive, non-toxic, and complementary ways of preventing and treating breast cancer. Her book, *The Complete Natural Medicine Guide to Breast Cancer*, is a source of hope and guidance for women the world over. It includes suggestions on supplementation alongside conventional treatment, as well as recommendations on how to minimize or even reverse the ravages of chemotherapy and radiation. Sat Dharam's gentle manner and vast knowledge attract countless women to her modest office in the small town of Owen Sound, Ontario. There, her Healing Arts Centre, a haven of calm, offers consultations, yoga, meditation, and other interventions that promote well-being.

Consulting with Sat Dharam and following her regime helped me to regain some feeling of control over my health. It gave me hope that I could find my way back to the sense of health and well-being I had enjoyed before I embarked on a conventional course of treatment for breast cancer. I only wish I had come across Sat Dharam and her important work when I was first diagnosed. Lori was lucky enough to have known Sat Dharam and her work when she was diagnosed with breast cancer. At the time of this interview, Lori remained in good health and attributed much of this to following Sat Dharam's protocol for breast cancer treatment.

Naturopathy
Naturopathy is a system of medicine based on helping the body to heal itself through detoxification, strengthening areas of weakness and the use of natural substances and non-invasive therapies.[7]

Sat Dharam, how did you become interested in working with women with breast cancer?

When I lived in Toronto in my twenties, a woman I knew had breast cancer and sought both conventional and alternative treatments. Her death made me realize that there was a need for a more systematic approach, so I began to think about and collect pieces that could be part of a program for women, first to prevent breast cancer and then to recover from and manage it. I taught workshops and lectured, and these eventually became the foundation for my book. I graduated in 1989 from the Naturopathic College, and since my thirties I've been treating people with all cancers, including a significant number of women with breast cancer.

What do you think are important precipitating factors for women with breast cancer?

Breast cancer is multifactorial. Oncologists often say we don't know why people develop breast cancer. I believe we do know why, and while it's not 100 percent certain, we need to do our best to identify those reasons for each woman. Factors, which I've listed in my book, include environmental toxins, hormonal imbalances, taking the pill at a young age, hormone replacement therapy, dietary factors, liver toxicity and

---

7   Kaur, S. D. (2003). *The Complete Natural Medicine Guide to Breast Cancer*. Toronto, ON: Robert Rose, p. 12.

the chronic constipation that contributes to it, fungal infections, issues in the mouth like amalgam fillings and root canal infections, spiritual factors, and genetic susceptibilities. Then there is the emotional factor. I think cancer happens when trauma hasn't been expressed and it's held in the body, especially when it relates to injustice, grief, and divorce. It helps for a woman to express that and heal from it. If we identify some of these triggers, women will feel empowered to do things to reverse them. I also believe that the breast cancer epidemic is not simply one woman's disease. It is our collective responsibility to reverse the causes of breast cancer by living sustainably, treading lightly on the earth, and refraining from poisoning the soil, water, and air.

When should a woman with breast cancer consult you?

Women come to me at different stages, and I support them at every stage — whether it is before or after surgery, before or after radiation, before or after chemotherapy, or after conventional therapies have been completed to prevent a recurrence. It's so much better if a woman comes to me before radiation and chemotherapy because there is so much that can be done naturally to help them through these treatments. If she comes after chemo and radiation, however, I do everything I would've done earlier, but not all of the damage is reversible. About 90 percent of the damage from chemo can be undone with naturopathic interventions.

What do you think about surgery for breast cancer?

I always recommend removing the tumour with surgery, though in two cases we got rid of it with topical salves. But even if the tumour load is gone, there are almost always some cancer cells circulating in the blood. Cancer is hard to get rid of because cancer cells have a life of their own — they don't die. If there are some cells left in the blood, then you can deal with them with naturopathic medicine. You need to be diligent for the rest of your life, and at least for five to ten years use supplements and a rigorous program to prevent recurrence. It takes about three years to get a woman on track, so I like to work with women over at least a three-year program.

What do you think about chemotherapy and radiation?

I don't have a black-and-white approach to chemotherapy and radiation, but they are often prescribed when people don't need them. I know that in the future there will be more tailoring of chemotherapy as to who receives it and what type.

If a woman comes to you during chemotherapy, what can you offer her?

If a woman comes to me during chemotherapy or radiation, I can give her herbs, mushrooms, and antioxidants to reduce the free radical load and keep her immune system as strong as possible during the treatments, thereby protecting her for later in life. Medical doctors say don't take anything during chemo, but that's ridiculous. The patients are stressed out about what to do, so I tell them to look at my website and make up their minds based on the studies cited there. Antioxidants can minimize the side effects and improve on the effects of chemo. But chemo drugs are carcinogens, and cancer could return due to free radical damage.

What can you do to protect women during radiation?

I believe the damage done by radiation is worse than the damage done by chemo. Women should be protected during radiation by taking more herbs, supplements, and antioxidants. Miso, kelp, and vitamin C will help eliminate radioactive molecules so they don't cause more damage. I'm very careful about the benefits of radiation versus the risks. I'm not saying not to do radiation, but some women die of heart and lung problems related to radiation.

What recommendations would you give regarding diet for women with breast cancer?

All the research I do tells me women with breast cancer need a plant-based diet. This includes foods that help reverse breast cancer, like flax seeds, organic soy, turmeric, garlic, rosemary, and members of the brassica family such as broccoli sprouts and cauliflower. We need to consume low-glycemic foods, increase our fibre, and cut out sugar.

High glycemic foods will cause high blood levels of insulin (and IGF-1) which causes increased fat storage. This causes increased estrogen, which combined with IGF-1, promotes breast cancer.[8]

If you eat sugar, meat, cheese, and other things that are risk factors, it's more likely you will have a recurrence. It's also important to buy organic.

What is your protocol for supplementation?
The body needs a lot of support to fight cancer because cancer can recur easily, so you need a rigorous routine with supplements as well as diet for the first five to ten years. This should include:
- curcumin [found in turmeric]
- NAC [N-acetylcysteine, a nutritional supplement]
- flax, indole-3-carbinol [found in cruciferous vegetables]
- fish oil
- flax seed oil

On my website, MammAlive.net, I list the top ten supplements with antioxidants, which include:
- grape seed extract
- CoQ10
- vitamin C
- mushrooms (reishi, coriolus, shiitake, and maitake)
- kelp

I use a variety of supplements to give women a lot of ammunition to prevent a recurrence. I test the effectiveness of supplementation with urine and blood tests in the US and Canada. Though it seems like I prescribe a lot of supplements, the numbers that come back from the labs show that the body is using almost all of them. While I think a woman is at risk for the rest of her life, if there is no recurrence in ten years, then it's likely that what has been done has worked and perhaps she can be less rigorous with supplements while maintaining the same lifestyle.

---

8   Kaur, S. D. (2003). *The Complete Natural Medicine Guide to Breast Cancer*. Toronto, ON: Robert Rose, p. 230.

What testing do you recommend for heavy metal overload in the body?

Though we can test for PCBs and pesticides, I assume they are in everybody and that women need to detox. One of the best ways to get rid of the heavy metal overload in the body is to sweat it out. My best estimate, given my testing on small groups of people and how much time it takes to get rid of 90 percent of environmental chemicals, is that you need about 150 hours in the sauna. This will also help to cut down the risk of recurrence. Additionally, there is a strong link between cancer and low-grade bacterial infections in the mouth generated by, for instance, amalgam fillings and root canals. You can evaluate infection in the jawbone or root canal tooth using MRI (magnetic resonance imaging) or cavitat (ultrasound), and can remove amalgam fillings. Many metals are estrogenic so they must be removed. You can test for the presence of metals with urine tests.

What about hormone testing to determine interventions to prevent recurrences?

Hormone testing is important. Insulin-like growth factor (IGF) is the strongest hormonal growth factor in breast cancer recurrence, followed by insulin, then estrogen. IGF shows up in the blood, but medical doctors don't usually check for it. I use Neuroscience Lab to check saliva levels of estriol, estradiol, and estrone, and Rocky Mountain Labs for urine testing to check the ratio between two estrogen metabolites, C2 (beneficial estrogen metabolites) and C16 (harmful estrogen metabolites). For estrogen metabolite ratios, you want to have lots of C2 and little C16. If that's the case, I know the liver is working well to break down estrogen in a healthy way. If the ratio is unfavourable, then I know I have to increase NAC, probiotics, curcumin, and fibre so the liver can handle estrogen better.

Estrogen's delicate balance

Estrogen comprises estrone (E1), estradiol (E2), and estriol (E3). Estradiol and estrone promote growth, and estriol stops growth, so they need to be in balance for optimal health.

What about the significance of blood stickiness, iron and ferritin levels, iodine levels, and tumour markers in preventing recurrences?

You need to keep the blood thin so there is no clumping, because the stickier the blood, the more likely it is that metastasis might occur. Therefore, measuring stickiness of blood with fibrinogen and fibrin d-dimers is important. You also need to look for signs of inflammation in the body, which will push cancer to grow faster, so we need to check for markers like C-reactive protein. High iron levels make people more susceptible to cancer, so keep iron low. Ferritin levels should be at about 90. One in nine people have hemochromatosis, an iron storage problem that increases a woman's breast cancer risk[9]. Women past menopause are much more susceptible to cancer, so that's another thing to look for. I also test vitamin D levels and do iodine loading tests in a few people, since there's a link between breast cancer and iodine. It's important to check tumour markers and repeat them annually. CEA and CA15-3 are the main ones.

What do you regard as the best tests to perform to get an overview of how the body is functioning and where to intervene for optimal health?

The ION profile blood and urine test is a fantastic test, though expensive. It is a total metabolic and nutritional test that looks at antioxidants, essential fatty acid levels, mineral status, liver detox pathways, cellular detox pathways, fungal or bacterial overload in the gut, strength of the heart, risk factors for the heart, and a few cancer markers. It helps me to fine-tune the nutritional status of the person. In two women with no suspicion of symptoms, I found out from this

---

9   Osborne, N. J., Gurrin, L. C., Allen, K. J., Constantine, C. C., Delatycki, M. B., McLaren, C. E., … English, D. R. (2010). HFE C282Y homozygotes are at increased risk of breast and colorectal cancer. *Hepatology 51*(4), 1311-1318. https://doi.org/10.1002/hep.23448

test they had an overwhelming fungal overload in the gut. It's good to do this test annually.

What kinds of tests could be done by the conventional health care system initially to improve on cancer treatment?

Firstly, if chemo is used, there should be more analysis of the tumour itself during and after surgery to determine which chemo works to kill the tumour. The tumour sensitivity test will determine that. It's good they are doing oncotype testing more routinely now to show who is more likely to have a recurrence and benefit from chemo.

Secondly, there could also be routine testing of breast cancer cells for infectious organisms. There is a study showing that 30 percent of breast cancer tumours have Epstein-Barr virus, and it's possible that a virus, not necessarily Epstein-Barr, turns on breast cancer genes and causes cancer[10,11,12,13]. Similarly, if a woman has infections in her teeth, she may need antifungal or antibacterial treatment to deal with the bacteria.

Thirdly, with respect to environmental toxins, it would be relatively simple to run a breast cancer tumour through a screen for toxins to

10   Huo, Q., Zhang, N., & Yang, Q. (2012). Epstein Barr virus infection and sporadic breast cancer risk: A meta-analysis. *PLOS ONE 7*(2). https://doi.org/10.1371/journal.pone.031656

11   Bonnet, M., Guinebretiere, J-M., Kremmer, E., Grunewald, V., Benhamou, E., Contesso, G., & Joab, I. (1999). Detection of Epstein-Barr virus in invasive breast cancers. *Journal of the National Cancer Institute 91*(16), 1376-1381. https://doi.org/10.1093/jnci/91.16.1376

12   Luqmani, Y., & Shousha, S. (1995). Presence of Epstein-Barr virus in breast carcinoma. *International Journal of Oncology 6*(4), 899-903. https://doi.org/10.3892/ijo.6.4.899

13   Lawson, J. S., Salmon, B., & Glen, W. K. (2018). Oncogenic viruses and breast cancer: Mouse mammary tumor virus (MMTV), bovine leukemia virus (BLV), human papilloma virus (HPV) and Epstein-Barr virus (EBV). *Frontiers in Oncology 8*(1). https://doi.org/10.3389/fonc.2018.00001

determine what toxic substances it has in it and compare them to benign breast tumours. Then, for example, I would suggest 150 hours in the sauna or other methods to get rid of the toxic chemicals. At present, it is not acknowledged that environmental toxins are related to breast cancer.

Fourthly, hormonal testing is crucial. Other than progesterone and estrogen testing, very few patients get enough done to see what's driving the cancer. We need to test everyone for blood sugar, IGF, and insulin levels. Some conventional doctors are using metformin now to prevent cancer recurrence in women who have already been treated for breast cancer, rather than recommending dietary change. I believe we should go back to the cause, which means fixing the diet that raises the blood sugar levels in the first place.

What is your opinion of adjuvant treatments like tamoxifen?

Tamoxifen can be helpful in preventing recurrence in estrogen receptor-positive [ER-positive] patients, but it has known side effects, including other cancers, such as uterine cancer, and blood clots. I think a number of well-designed studies are needed to compare the effectiveness of tamoxifen with flax seeds and soy, and to decide if, as the evidence suggests, flax seeds and soy are better — though they aren't money-makers.

What about aromatase inhibitors?

Aromatase inhibitors (AI's) can work well for some women, and they're not carcinogenic like tamoxifen. I don't have a problem recommending AIs. But the side effects, like joint pain and loss of bone mineral density (particularly in the jaw), can interfere with quality of life for some people. A dose of 50,000 IU per week of vitamin D will reverse most of the side effects, and the bone density loss can be managed with other naturopathic medications. AIs can inhibit fat cells' production of estrogen, but their utility is limited because you want to manage the blood sugar and IGF at the same time. We could be using natural supplements like flax seeds, soy, zinc, and grape seed extract, which act like AIs. We should also be doing studies to compare their effectiveness.

Aromatase is an enzyme that produces estrogen.

I keep hearing of women who are on tamoxifen and aromatase inhibitors who have a recurrence when they stop at the five- or seven-year mark.

Yes, that's right. It's common for medical doctors to take women off tamoxifen or AIs after five years, and women get freaked out. The therapy is incomplete and they need to continue to manage and protect against the estrogen with indole-3-carbinol, flax seeds, soy, and an overall naturopathic regime.

If you can do that at the five-year mark, can you do it from the start without tamoxifen?

Absolutely, I believe you can do that from the start. But we need comparative studies to prove it. I have a lot of patients for whom it has been fifteen to twenty years since they had cancer, and they feel better than they have ever felt. My experience tells me that women with a history of breast cancer can live well and die of something else if they follow my program. There are a few exceptions, such as if something is missed or the genetics are stacked against them. For instance, if the oncotype test shows you have all twenty-one genes, it's difficult to prevent recurrence.

The oncotype test analyzes the activity of twenty-one different genes, which will help determine whether you are likely to have a recurrence.

If a woman has limited financial resources, what are the most important things she can do?

Firstly, if I have to choose, diet is very important, and it's a good place to start. Sugar feeds cancer. A mainly vegan diet with a high percentage of fruits and vegetables, and with nuts as a protein source, will inhibit cancer. We can do a lot with diet alone.

Secondly, 3,000 IUs of vitamin D3 daily is very important for decreasing breast cancer risk by about 60 percent.[14] The liver and kidneys need support, so increase bowel movements to three to four per day - that lowers the estrogen levels and the overall toxic load in the body. Use a sauna to sweat out toxins. Another simple thing is to take 4,000 mg of vitamin C daily to help pull out heavy metals. This decreases the risk of breast cancer recurrence by decreasing the load of toxins in the body.

Thirdly, one could do an environmental detox. Eliminate plastic, avoid chlorine pools, use organic cleansers, and eat organic foods. My book includes a four-page list of all the things that are related to breast cancer and ways to reverse them.

Finally, I think a big factor is stress. We need to balance our stress with meditation and exercise, and to engage in self-care so that busyness doesn't overwhelm our lives.

Sugar and breast cancer surgery

All sugar that is taken into the body is broken down by the body into glucose. Glucose can cause secretion of lactic acid, which triggers a drop in the body's alkalinity. This can provide a favourable environment in which cancer metastases occurs. Because cancer cells love sugar, it is usual for a sugar dye to be injected into the breast lymphatic system prior to surgery for breast cancer. The dye will attach to any malignant cells in the lymphatic system, highlighting tumours along the way. An article in the Canadian newspaper *The National Post* reported that the appetite of cancer cells for sugar is three times that of normal cells.[15]

---

14   Cunningham, D., Gilchrist, N. L., Cowan, R. A., Forrest, J. F., McArdle, C. S., & Soukop, M. (1985). Alfacalcidol as a modulator of growth of low grade non-Hodgkin's lymphomas. *British Medical Journal 291*(6503), 1153. Retrieved from https://www.ncbi.nlm.nih.gov/pmc/articles/PMC1417870/

15   MacDougal, J. (2014, February 1). What does cancer eat? Sugar, mostly and other lessons from my dinner with a professor of

What kind of success have you had with your protocol?

Out of about one hundred and fifty patients, two patients didn't do so well after following my program. I don't have studies to prove it, but I would say that even though I've had patients who have had recurrence and died, I can put a finger on what caused that to happen.

What kind of relationship would you like to see between naturopathic doctors and medical doctors?

We need a protocol that bridges both parties. Despite the fact that patients are seeing alternative practitioners anyway, it'll be a long time before those bridges are built in Ontario because medical doctors are blinded by medical research. They view issues narrowly, one thing at a time, rather than broadly. As a consequence of this lack of co-operation, patients are forced to become intermediaries in the conflicts between the naturopathic and conventional worlds. This causes them more stress and is not acceptable at this time in a breast cancer patient's life.

---

pathology. *National Post*. Retrieved from https://nationalpost.com/life/jane-macdougall-what-does-cancer-eat-sugar-mostly-and-other-lessons-from-my-dinner-with-a-professor-of-pathology

CHAPTER 5

Dr. Alvin Pettle, Gynecologist

When Lori was first diagnosed with breast cancer, she had recently consulted Dr. Alvin Pettle, an integrative gynecologist. Lori considers herself lucky that her cancer diagnosis coincided with that meeting, since Dr. Pettle met her terror with warmth and understanding. Dr. Pettle was able to suggest safe hormonal interventions for someone with breast cancer, as well as guide her to other like-minded professionals. Dr. Pettle's strategies for women with breast cancer have included correcting their hormonal imbalances while also paying attention to other factors such as diet and supplementation. His program illustrates that treatments with few side effects can be obtained outside of mainstream medicine and can be successful for many people.

Dr. Pettle trained in obstetrics and gynaecology at Mount Sinai Hospital in Toronto. He was one of the few obstetricians in North America performing the gentle birthing technique called Leboyer. However, by the time Lori met Dr. Pettle, he had abandoned his thriving obstetrics practice, disappointed that even one of the best medical educations in Canada had failed to consider important preventative health matters such as diet and spirituality. He went on to develop the only medical practice in the country that worked with bio-identical hormones in the 1990s. These hormones, which have the same molecular structure as the body's own hormones, are a safer alternative to synthetic hormones in women whose own supply has become depleted with age. Eight years after Lori's contact with Dr.

Pettle, I found myself in his waiting room, which felt like a private living room and a tranquil retreat. There, a flood of women seeking out his natural interventions for treating and managing breast cancer, menopause, and hormonal imbalances gathered. Dr. Pettle continues to dispense his immense knowledge, skills, and flexible views regarding interventions with great courage, despite the fact that on numerous occasions he has dealt with the disapproval of his medical colleagues regarding his views on bio-identical hormonal management in women. Dr. Pettle's passion and generosity were a source of inspiration for me as I struggled to find my way forward in the wake of my own cancer experience.

Dr. Pettle, what do you believe causes breast cancer?

A woman's path to breast cancer is multifactorial. It's a result of the wrong person because of their genetics, being in the wrong place, because of the influence of environmental factors, at the wrong time — that is, where we stand in relation to society and evolution. Firstly, genes can be a cause. The BRCA gene mutation is the main one, and it affects mostly descendants of Ashkenazi Jews, but there are many others yet to be identified. My grandmother, my mother, and her two sisters died of breast cancer. That was genetic. You've now got to look at every daughter of those people, because everyone who is a descendant is at a high risk. For example, usually Jewish people marry within the race, and it weakens the race because recessive genes marrying recessive genes eventually become dominant.

And then there is diet. If a sister and mother have breast cancer, maybe they're eating the same things and their diet isn't great. But something similar that they are putting into their system, in combination with environmental toxins and their genetic makeup, causes breast cancer.

Thirdly, anxiety and fear create stress and hormone imbalance. As soon as there is an imbalance in hormones, the whole body becomes aware of it. I really believe that if a woman has breast cancer, somewhere along the line a hormonal disorder of cortisol has occurred. That hormonal imbalance can take root early on in a woman's development, when she is around the age of twelve, or even earlier when, one year prior to menses, she develops thelarche — that is breast development. I think it can begin when you first realize you are a woman, and you either feel you are comfortable with men and trust them, or you worry that there is danger out there and that something inappropriate will happen. That anxiety causes stress, which eventually causes the hormone DHEA (dehydroepiandrosterone) to become depleted. Another risk factor is menstruating past fifty-five. You and your health care provider need to be aware of this risk and monitor it.

How do you work with newly diagnosed breast cancer patients?
When I see a person initially, and they already have a diagnosis of breast cancer, my role is to co-captain with them. I work almost in the background, considering where they are in the allopathic world that is, what treatment choices they have made in the conventional medical system. I give them additional medical information, and support their decisions. I encourage them not to worry about me, but to feel free to say anything they would like about their situation that elicits a feeling of comfort, and the truth becomes more apparent about which course of treatment, including chemo and radiation, is right for them. Unfortunately, they are caught up in a triangle, and their final decision is influenced by the pressure they get from the conventional medical world, the information they get from me, and their own feelings. So when a woman comes to me and says that they removed a lump along with her lymph nodes, and they want to give her chemo and radiation, but she doesn't want to do it, I'll support her wishes and say, don't do it. I think it's important that if a doctor senses fear in a patient's eyes about chemotherapy or radiation, then he or she should be able to say, you know what? It may not make much difference anyway. On the other hand, I've had patients come in here and say they want a mastectomy or chemotherapy or radiation, and when I ask them how they feel about that and they say okay, I say don't go against your instincts. Stay with that, and when you are done, we'll talk again. If you tell a person you have to do this or that, you are augmenting their stress. I think life is shades of grey, not

black and white, and there has to be an elasticity on the part of the doctor. That means the patient needs to come up with answers with the physician's approval and support. Unfortunately, that elasticity is too often not a part of the allopathic program.

What do you think are important ingredients in preventing a recurrence in breast cancer patients?

If someone got cancer once, and you change the milieu, the soil in which the cancer grew in the first place, you can possibly prevent a recurrence of the cancer. There was a guy who used to be head of the Canadian College of Naturopathic Medicine who said that you can't grow daisies in cement. What he meant was you need to change a person's whole attitude towards nutrition, exercise, water, living, loving. So I try to understand that person's perception of things, her diet, what she eats, and her sleep patterns. Then the system must be cleaned out — in particular the liver — to get her digestion going. Drinking half her weight in water (one ounce of water for every two pounds she weighs) will help to do this. Then there's the emotional factor, which as I mentioned earlier is also important. It includes her sexuality, her comfort with men, and her relationship with her parents. Sometimes I need to go back in time with someone else, perhaps a psychotherapist, a naturopath, or a homeopath, to see if this woman has been harmed or injured. A person who has been raped or abused may or may not deal with the trauma, and that decision can have a positive or negative impact on her health. There's a theory that says the left side of the body relates to issues with the mother, the right side with the father. Sometimes, when the illness occurs on one or other side of the body, it can inform us.

Disorders of the hormonal system related to cortisol need to be dealt with. Anxiety and stress cause elevated cortisol, which lowers the hormone DHEA and over time lowers one's defences. This is one of the biggest factors causing breast cancer. In the factory that most people go through for breast cancer treatment, you can have a good outcome and come out of it. But once you're out alive, be passionate about things, as the Greeks said, and get back to normal but not the normal from before. You've got to change some things, which takes us back to the soil, the milieu that the cancer grows in.

What do you think of mammograms?

Mammograms- that's a complicated question. It was decided long ago by conventional medical doctors to use mammography for screening, but it's not a screening device. A mass can be picked up on a mammogram, but not a diagnosis of cancer. It's a device that should be used when an appropriate physical and genetic history is taken and that history suggests that the patient is at a high risk for breast cancer, because of, for example, fibrocystic breasts, hormone replacement therapy, diet, or genetics. Doctors have to mammograph one hundred people to find a few cases of cancer. While it is important to find those few cases, it's best to do an educated mammogram using other benign instruments initially, because a mammogram crushes, irradiates, and traumatizes a breast. If men had to put their genitals under a machine like that, I believe they would have looked for another test a long time ago. So if I feel a mass in a patient's breast and she tells me she's had a normal mammogram, I'll look for more information. If she puts her hands up in the air and her breast indents, I need to know what it is. I usually know from an examination, the sense I have from palpating someone's breast, her history over the last five to ten years, and her own sense of it, when the mass has been sitting around for too long. For example, if I examine a woman who has a mass in her left breast at two o'clock and I don't like the mass, I might suggest a thermogram first. If she does a thermogram and at two o'clock on the left breast it's hot, which means there is inflammatory activity there, I'd like the opinion of a surgeon, so we biopsy it. Or alternatively I might go straight for the biopsy. In many cases it's cancer and the mammogram missed it, so mammograms aren't perfect either.

Can you do a biopsy without first doing a mammogram?

Sure you can. You can use an ultrasound or a thermogram. An ultrasound can help you decide whether a mammogram is necessary. On an ultrasound, fluid in fibrocystic breast lumps shows up black. If it feels cystic, I'd do an ultrasound and thermogram and then, if I have to, I'd do a mammogram. You still have to keep your license and not miss anything, but I've learned to be more elastic and use common sense. But a mass could be missed on an ultrasound, so it's a good idea to use it in conjunction with other tests. You can't rely on just one thing.

A thermogram is a tool that measures heat coming off a breast caused by increased blood flow and cellular activity.[16,17,18] You put your hands in cold water for a specified amount of time, to bring your overall body temperature down. While the blood vessels of normal tissue in the breast will cool down, tumour tissue remains hot. The heat sensing infrared scanners will detect the heat coming from the tumours and highlight this area on the screen.

By the way, a thermogram is a good preventive tool, but it's not perfect either because it can miss breast cancer. It's a benign diagnostic tool that adds to the information we need to do a biopsy, if necessary. Moreover, if you had thermogrammed a patient ten years earlier and it showed the patient had hot breasts, why wouldn't you counsel that person to become a vegetarian, as well as her sister and

16   Parisky, Y. R., Sardi, A., Hamm R., Hughes, K., Esserman, L., Rust, S., & Callahan, K. (2003). Efficacy of computerized infrared imaging analysis to evaluate mammographically suspicious lesions. *American Journal of Roentgenology, 180*(1), 263-269. https://doi.org/10.2214/ajr.180.1.1800263

17   Wishart, G. C., Campisi, M., Boswell, M., Chapman, D., Shackleton, V., Iddles, S., ... Britton, P. D. (2010) The accuracy of digital infrared imaging for breast cancer detection in women undergoing breast biopsy. *European Journal of Surgical Oncology,36*(6), 534-540. https://doi.org/10.1016/j.ejso.2010.04.003

18   Kolarić, D., Herceg, Z., Nola, I. A., Ramljak, V., Kulis, T., Holjevac, J. K., ... Antonini, S. (2013). Thermography – a feasible method for screening breast cancer? *Collegium Antropologicum, 37*(2), 583-8. Retrieved from https://www.ncbi.nlm.nih.gov/pubmed/23941007

her daughter? It could save that woman's life. What I mean is that the thermogram may have flagged an elevated risk in the family. This risk may be related to a genetic predisposition or to those other factors in families that we are not clear about that may predispose them to cancers such as breast cancer. If you counsel them to change their diet then at least they are being attentive to one factor that helps them to minimize their risk of getting this disease.

What is your opinion of MRIs?
I'm not an expert on MRIs, but I'm not sure I'd do so many MRIs, although sometimes they are necessary. If you are talking about doing an MRI, you have already seen something concerning on a mammogram and are expecting to confirm or disconfirm that finding.

You are aligned with surgery for breast cancer patients?
Yes, I'm okay with taking the mass in the breast out, and taking a sample of the sentinel node. If the cancer is in the nodes other interventions might be needed. A homeopath I know would say leave the lymph nodes but he doesn't have to keep a medical license; I do. And some people feel they've removed the cancer with surgery, so psychologically it's probably a good idea for them because that idea gives them hope. However, once there's a mass, all the other cells in the body know that the cancer was there. And if it's big enough to be a mass, it's no longer a few abnormal cells, and the question becomes why it's there in the first place. So we have to change more fundamental things or it may recur in another organ. By the way, we all have cancer cells, and when your immune system is working well, it mops them up. That's one of the things that DHEA does. That's what people have lost when their cortisol has been too high for too long. Stress opens the door to the house where cancer resides.

What do you think about chemotherapy and radiation?
Some people who decided not to take therapy are still alive, and some people who took therapy are no longer here. So who lives and who doesn't is a combination of multiple factors, which include being

informed and aware of what's happening to you, using your intuition about interventions and seeking out those that make sense to you, and having a positive attitude to life. But if a person has cancer in the lymph nodes, the whole body knows it has cancer. I remember a pathologist in one of our classes in medical school made the point that that the knowledge and awareness of cancer in one place in the body is likely known by every cell in the body. So I don't know if chemo would change anything. Probably chemotherapy and radiation are more destructive than anything else but maybe psychologically the person feels they've been treated completely and they're going to go on a new path; they've been to death's door and they will change their life, and maybe that will take them to the point where it will turn them around and they'll come back. I believe that in some cases you can reverse the mechanism by which it was made and stop the cancer by using means other than chemotherapy or radiation. For instance, you can use Myomins, herbs that are natural aromatase inhibitors, and detoxify the liver of estrone and estradiol so that the mass, which is dependent on estrogen, gets smaller.

You believe that excessive cortisol is a major contributing factor to breast cancer?

Yes, that's right. I don't think people get old and get cancer. I think people lose their immunity in this stressful world, their defences are down, and they are at high risk for cancer depending on their genetic makeup. By the time you are thirty, forty, or fifty, DHEA, one of the master hormones, is so low there is little immunity. If you look at every person who walks into my office, nine out of ten have high cortisol levels, little DHEA, and no immunity left. Our reproductive system is not programmed to go past fifty, and when the ovaries shut down during menopause, the adrenal glands need to take over. But if stress has depleted the adrenals and DHEA is low and cortisol high, the adrenals are unable to take over this function from the ovaries, and this further stresses the system. A stressed cell is a hypoxic [under-oxygenated] cell, and hypoxic cells can make mistakes in cell division; that is, multiply out of control with abnormal cells. Breast cancer risk is then elevated. Adrenal fatigue is at the root of cortisol production. I have found that DHEA drops under the tongue work best in replenishing depleted DHEA. The drops go into the circulatory system, the brain and the body then think they have made DHEA, and the cortisol level drops because the brain turns off ACTH — adrenal corticotropic hormone.[19,20] DHEA pills aren't effective because they go straight to the liver, which then converts it to the worst kind of estrogen, estrone, giving you a fatty liver. DHEA cream doesn't go through the skin fast enough. The dosage and absorption of the drops can be monitored with twenty-four-hour urine testing. Anybody who takes DHEA should take an aromatase inhibitor as well so that the DHEA is not converted into the bad estrogen, but rather into estriol, the good estrogen. DHEA is like anti-stress in a bottle. Some European studies have used vaginal (trans-mucosal) DHEA successfully. This will likely come to North America, if it hasn't already.

What is your opinion of tamoxifen and aromatase inhibitors?
I personally believe that tamoxifen has too many side effects to consider as an option. If you are going to stop the effects of estrogen overload, you need to use more specific medications. Estrogen can't be tagged as the villain. Estrogen comprises E1 (estrone), E2 (estradiol), and E3 (estriol). E1 and E2 are alpha stimulators and promote growth, E3 stops growth. You need to examine the composition of the estrogen and balance it. This will prevent an overload of the bad estradiol and estrone, both of which promote tumour growth. Estriol is administered vaginally and, if monitored, can work well to promote

---

19 Kalimi, M., Shafagoj, Y., Loria, R., Padgett, D., & Regelson, W. (1994) Anti-glucocorticoid effects of dehydroepiandrosterone (DHEA). *Molecular Cell Biochemistry, 131*(2), 99-104. Retrieved from https://link.springer.com/article/10.1007%2FBF00925945

20 Regelson, W., & Kalimi, M. (1994). Dehydroepiandrosterone (DHEA) - the Multifunctional Steroid. *Annals of New York Academy of Science, 719*(1), 564-75. https://doi.org/10.1111/j.1749-6632.1994.tb56860.x

a healthy balance of the hormone. It's also important to educate people about estrogen overload in their lives, including in nutrition and diet. It doesn't make sense to take tamoxifen and then drink a glass of milk, which has 300 milligrams of estrogen in it. Arimidex, an aromatase inhibitor, blocks estrogen receptors, so I feel it is appropriate in many cases.

If a woman with an estrogen receptor-positive cancer decides not to use tamoxifen or an aromatase inhibitor, are there other things she might do to manage the estrogen?

In a case of ER-positive cancer, I'd give her indole-3-carbinol and DIM supplements [active ingredients in cruciferous vegetables] because indole-3-carbinol and DIM ameliorate the effects of estrogen and eventually cause cancer cells to undergo apoptosis. Various supplements, including Myomins, help the liver rid itself of potent toxins, including potent estrogen, E1 (estrone) and E2 (estradiol). Cancer patients need to follow a diet similar to that of diabetics. I'd tell her to follow a mostly vegetarian diet and eat cruciferous vegetables (for example cabbage, cauliflower, broccoli) because they convert estrone to estriol. Eat hard fruits such as apples and pears, which are complex carbohydrates and are broken down into glucose at a slower rate. Fish is important because essential fatty acids which are found in fish but not in vegetables build necessary protein. Beans, quinoa, amaranth are all fine, but anything from a cow is not. Yogurt from goat's milk is fine. Pasta, breads, and rice, including whole wheat products and brown rice, still have hidden sugars. A woman with ER-positive cancer should drink half her body weight in ounces of water daily (for example, if she weighs 100 pounds she should drink 50 fluid ounces per day) to detoxify the liver. Regular exercise, and herbs such as milk thistle and dandelion, works well to cleanse the liver. Pancreatin helps the pancreas to detox and get rid of estrogen.

What kinds of hormonal interventions do you think a woman with breast cancer can safely use?

Contrary to what many people believe, there are no contraindications for using estriol with an estrogen positive cancer.[21,22] You want the good stuff — that is estriol — to bind to the receptors, so if you administer a small amount vaginally, you will improve your quality of life and protect against breast cancer. Once I've administered it, it's crucial to monitor it with an ultrasound of the uterus. If the lining is thinner than 5 millimetres in menopause, you have your estrogen under control. If the lining is too thick and bleeds, you take a sample and deal with that. The importance of estriol was demonstrated by a physician, Dr. Henry Lemon.[23] Over several decades, he studied the beneficial effects of estriol both in preventing and in managing breast cancer. In one of his studies, he administered estriol to twenty-eight women with breast cancer and metastases in the bone who had been told to go home and die. Their secondary cancers in the bone shrank, and 37 percent had total remission because the estriol was blocking the cancer rather than feeding it. That was almost forty years ago, but no one paid enough attention to his findings. Estriol has to be prescribed by a complementary physician; you can't get it from food.

The other crucial ingredient is progesterone. I'm in line with the late, brilliant Dr. John Lee who said the body may develop

---

21 Siteri, P. K. (2002, September). *Prospective study of estrogens during pregnancy and risk of breast cancer.* Presented at Department of Defense Breast Cancer Research Meeting, Berkley, CA.

22 Takahashi, K., Okada, M., Ozaki, T., Kurioka, H., Manabe, H., Kanasaki, H., & Miyazaki, K. (2000). Safety and efficacy of oestriol for symptoms of natural or surgically induced menopause. *Human Reproduction, 15*(5), 1028-1036. Retrieved from https://www.ncbi. nlm.nih.gov/pubmed/10783346

23 Lemon, H. M. (1987). Antimammary carcinogenic activity of 17-alpha-ethinyl estriol. *Cancer, 60*(12), 2873-2881. https://doi. org/10.1002/1097-0142(19871215)60:123.0.CO;2-B

progesterone-positive receptors to protect itself from estrogen.[24] When a woman ovulates, she produces progesterone. Progesterone is a great protector, and women who have had several pregnancies generally have a lower breast cancer risk. Progesterone is the body's natural anti-estrogen, and it counters the effect of adrenal imbalance by keeping estrogen in check.[25,26,27] Deficiency in this hormone leads to estrogen overload and ultimately breast cancer. I recommend both estriol and progesterone when administered under supervision and monitored with twenty-four hour urine testing to ensure that 20 percent of the estrogen content in her urine is estriol. This number is determined by dividing the estriol content in the urine by the estrone content and then adding the estradiol content. The final number should be greater than one. Estriol and progesterone will protect a woman from breast cancer by lowering her cortisol and also her bad estrogen. It will also rid her of dry vagina and sleep problems, and contribute to youthfulness. So, in my experience, if your cancer was progesterone-negative and you take progesterone cream, it will change your life and take you on the next part of your journey.

24   Lee, J. R., Zava, D., & Hopkins, V. (2005). *What your doctor may not tell you about breast cancer: How hormone balance can help save your life*. New York, NY: Warner Books, pp. 132-134.

25   Formby, B., & Wiley, T. S. (1998). Progesterone inhibits growth and induces apoptosis in breast cancer cells: Inverse effects on Bcl-2 and p53. *Annals of Clinical and Laboratory Science, 28*(6), 360-369. Retrieved from https://www.ncbi.nlm.nih.gov/pubmed/9846203

26   Dugan, S., & Sciopione, A. (2006, April). Progesterone misconceptions. *Life Extension Magazine*. Retrieved from https://www.lifeextension.com/magazine/2006/4/report_progesterone/Page-02

27   Stein, D. C. (2006). The case for progesterone. *Annals of the New York Academy of Science, 1052*, 152-169. https://doi.org/10.1196/annals.1347.011

How do you deal with the conventional medical community's reaction to people like you, who have the courage to practise outside the box?

You create a new box. Maybe it's related to the confidence that comes when you provide wellness and care. If you have the courage of your convictions, you'll stick by what you think is right. And usually right wins. It's about re-thinking things as they evolve. Synthetic oral hormone replacement therapy (HRT) is a good example of this. It was used by so many doctors for so many years, ultimately with questionable outcomes. People who have the ideas first are usually thought to be manic or mad, but the truth ultimately prevails.

> **The Women's Health Initiative and HRT**
> In 1991, the National Institutes of Health launched the Women's Health Initiative across the US. This was a study, involving more than 16,000 women, to determine whether estrogen —with or without progestin — helped women with menopausal symptoms. The study was stopped prematurely in 2002 because it found that HRT was associated with an increased risk of breast cancer, heart disease, stroke, and urinary incontinence.[28]

What is your success rate with women who accept your recommended interventions?

In the twenty-five years I've been working this way, I would say that to my knowledge, in patients of mine who were diagnosed with breast cancer while under my care, there would be fewer than a dozen who succumbed prematurely to the cancer.

---

28   Gurney, E. P., Nachtigall, M. J., Nachtigall, L. E., & Naftolin, F. (2014). The women's health initiative trial and related studies: 10 years later: A clinician's view. *Journal of Steroid Biochemistry and Molecular Biology, 142,* 4-11. https://doi.org/10.1016/j.jsbmb.2013.10.009

CHAPTER 6

Dr. Alex Mostovoy, Homeopath

When Lori was first diagnosed, Dr. Pettle sent her to consult with a homeopath, Dr. Alex Mostovoy. Dr. Mostovoy administered various remedies to help Lori with wound care and healing, a course she followed over the next year. Dr. Mostovoy, who completed a four-year post-graduate training program at the Homeopathic College of Canada, is the only board-certified clinical thermographer in Canada. He pioneered the use of breast thermography in Toronto and educates physicians about the benefits of breast thermography as a screening tool. Dr. Mostovoy was very gracious when we met and put much thought into conveying his views on cancer treatments. He was baffled by the rigidity of the current standard of care offered by allopathic medicine for breast and other cancers, and likens the prevailing protocol to a military model stuck in the Middle Ages. He believes that fruitless search-and-destroy missions to find the cancer leave countless casualties in their wake, predisposing a person to more medical problems later, including other cancers.

Dr. Mostovoy, what is homeopathy?
Homeopathy is a two-hundred-year-old treatment that has barely changed since its inception. It cures like with like and is individualized for each patient.

Homeopathy also involves using small amounts of a substance that would cause harm in larger amounts.

It also considers emotional health in its evaluation and treatment, and is therefore time-consuming to practise. There are about three thousand substances in the homeopathic pharmacopeia, and various substances encourage certain physical and emotional symptoms to emerge in the patient. Many of the symptoms, sensations, and themes that emerge are chronicled in the homeopathic pharmacopeia, and are of much interest when I work with a person.

What do you believe are the causative factors of breast cancer?
Only 10 percent of cancers are genetic; 90 percent are environmental. By environment, I don't mean just pollutants, but the overall environment: diet, lifestyle, medications, and emotional health.[29,30] The greatest ecological disaster may not be just polluted oceans or air, but the effect of environmental pollutants on the hormonal systems of both women and men. Many breast cancers are related to women's reactions to estrogen. Some people who have had cancer have also had mononucleosis or Epstein-Barr virus, so their practitioners should test for these viruses more closely.

Emotions are crucial, because the way you think affects you on a biochemical level. For example, when people are depressed, they are much more susceptible to viral infections. So if we view human beings as psycho-emotional, bioenergetic, biophysical beings, we are getting

---

29 Anand, P., Kunnumakkara, A. B., Sundaram, C., Harikumar, K. B., Tharakan, S. T., Lai, O. S., ... Aggarwal, B. B. (2008). Cancer is a preventable disease that requires major lifestyle changes. *Pharmaceutical Research, 25*(9), 2097-2116. https://doi.org/10.1007/s11095-008-9661-9

30 Mezzetti, M., La Vecchia, C., Decarli, A., Boyle, P., Talamini, R., & Franceschi, S. (1998). Population attributable risk for breast cancer: diet, nutrition, and physical exercise. *Journal of the National Cancer Institute, 90*(5), 389-394. Retrieved from https://www.ncbi.nlm.nih.gov/pubmed/9498489

closer to addressing the individual on a holistic level and, therefore, are more likely to resolve the disease.

How do you work with breast cancer patients?

We all have cancer cells and our system is constantly dealing with them, but we need to understand at what point they grew out of control because our system could no longer deal with them. People don't just wake up with cancer; it's been in the making for nine or ten years. So I have to become familiar with what kind of cancer the patient has, who they are, what their dreams and weak points are, their role in their family, and the stress this might have caused them. Then I can understand what brought this patient to the point of disease. That's where I start. For example — a simple analogy — if somebody's root canal was infected twenty years ago but never treated, it can fester and affect the lymphatics, create neurotoxin waste products, and shut down neuro tumour suppression genes, and breast cancer may develop. It's possible someone could go through conventional or unconventional therapy with breast cancer but still not address the root cause. The way I tackle it to effect a cure is to take the body through the disease process in reverse. I do this by shifting the disease from the chronic, to the sub-acute, to the acute level, or in other words, peeling off layer by layer in reverse occurrence. This way the symptoms can be more easily treated and the patient can regain her health.

What do you think about conventional treatments?

Cancer is a very political and emotional thing, and conventional practitioners have deluded themselves into believing their way is the only way. But the invasiveness and total suppression of the immune system in modern treatments of cancer doesn't make sense to me. Measuring whether the tumour is shrinking or getting bigger addresses only one of many variables. I don't believe one rule fits all. There are different types of breast cancers (for example, ductal carcinoma in situ [DCIS] and lobular carcinoma) and different stages of the disease process. The different cancers have different causes, which need to be more carefully considered. Eighty percent of eighty-year-old women have

DCIS when they die, but die of something else. Probably 50 percent of fifty-year-olds have DCIS but are not symptomatic. But the majority of people are overwhelmed with fear when they are diagnosed with cancer because it's very confusing out there. If they even consider other options, often their friends, family, and physicians will say, "What, you're not doing chemo?" They then succumb to their fear and continue with the conventional form of treatment. Nevertheless, I've had patients who have gone the conventional route for breast cancer and are doing great, and I've had patients with huge tumours in their breasts who have not gone the conventional route and now live well and have full lives.

Common types of breast cancer

Ductal carcinoma in situ (DCIS)
A non-invasive cancer that has not spread beyond the milk ducts, considered by some to be "Stage Zero."

Invasive ductal carcinoma
An invasive cancer that starts in the milk ducts.

Invasive lobular carcinoma
An invasive cancer that starts in the milk glands or lobules, and spreads to the surrounding tissue.

Let's say a person is frightened and does follow a conventional route for treatment. How effective can your work be if she has gone this route?

My strategy is to stimulate the immune system, whereas the conventional system uses methods that suppress it. If this is the route the patient is taking, I take a back seat and support them by easing the side effects — the nausea, the hair loss — and work with them on emotional issues. My role under these circumstances changes from being the primary caregiver to being supportive.

Can any of your interventions reverse the damage of chemotherapy or radiation?

I can help a patient recover and rebuild faster from chemo or radiation, and can lessen the effects as she is going through it, but I can't reverse the damage done to the DNA by chemo and radiation. However, we are dynamic human beings with an incredible ability to rejuvenate and regain health. Therefore, damage done by chemo and radiation can in some cases be reversed, but that depends on many variables. This is medicine, not mathematics.

What interventions do you recommend in order to prevent recurrence?

If we can determine what brought the person to this level and address it, we can lower the chances of recurrence because there is no longer a reason for the cancer to be there. If I can help someone to eat well, lose extra weight, and exercise, it lowers their risk of recurrence. If they're stuck on some emotional issue, overcoming trauma will reduce the risk of recurrence.

What do you think about tamoxifen and aromatase inhibitors?

Aromatase inhibitors interfere with a biochemical process. Those who use them assume that by knocking out this or that enzyme, they're correcting the problem. I think they are off the mark because they don't know what the problem is that they are attempting to correct. Any interference with the biological process will have side effects. For example, if someone converts good estrogen to bad estrogen or testosterone to estradiol, you can slow down the rate of growth by prescribing AI's or tamoxifen. But that conversion is there for a reason, and by blocking out bad things, you also block out good things. Instead I think that aiding the body in the natural process of healing can be more helpful. People should be encouraged to manage their diet to deal with the problem. Coffee, alcohol, and cheese convert testosterone to estradiol. It would be much healthier for the person to sit down with experts in nutrition and work out a good diet. By intervening with chemicals, we create an imbalance on different levels.

I like to work with the person, not against them, because the only true healing is self-healing.

If a woman has limited financial means, what should she do, given that alternative practitioners aren't covered under provincial health insurance?
I've never rejected a patient because they can't pay. If they have difficulties I'll say, "pay what you can." I realize some people are struggling because the disease has knocked them out.

What advice would you give to a woman who's just been diagnosed with breast cancer?
People succumb to fear. It's best to not make decisions when you are fearful or angry.

You said that in a majority of cases you don't interfere, but play more of a supportive role. Why?
I see myself as an instrument of healing, so I guide the patient, who needs to accept responsibility for the healing process in order for us to proceed. However, I don't control the outcome, and I don't feel that if they don't do it my way they are doomed. So I don't try to convince people, in contrast to an oncologist who might say, "if you don't do it my way you'll die." Even if they do die, he just says that what he did was "standard of care." Each person needs to tune into her own intuition and do what she feels is right. I see people as individuals who require individual approaches — every case is unique.

What do you think about surgery?
In many cases if we cut things out, we speed up the process of recurrence elsewhere in the body in a more aggressive way. What I mean is that the body is always trying to be in a state of homeostasis. The tumour manifestation is an expression of a much deeper process; therefore eliminating the tumour with surgery (and doing nothing else) does not address the underlying cause of the disease. In my opinion, this may trigger a metastatic process in the organism in some cases.

That's the way the body works. If you have a pimple and cut it out, you don't eliminate the cause of the pimple. A tumour, like a pimple, is a symptom of the disease, not the disease itself. The body is giving you a clue that something is off. If you go after the clue by cutting out the lump instead of dealing with the problem on a systemic level, the body might give you a second message in a slightly stronger tone — that is, with a second growth that is a little more aggressive.

What do you think about chemotherapy?
Chemo kills a lot of cells in the hope that it will get the ones we want to kill. In early stages of cancer, the organism is still strong enough to resist and survive assault. But in late stages, the organism may not survive; it's weakened. Eventually chemo can shrink the tumour, but the patient dies six months later because it's irrevocably weakened the immune system.

Do you believe that your interventions have a better outcome than chemotherapy and radiation?
There are so many different factors. We need to understand where we are in the disease's process, and that's very difficult to assess because we don't have the technology to measure it. We have staging processes; we measure tumour size — but in the end, it's a primitive way of looking at it, and in my opinion isn't an accurate measure. If it's in a very early stage, the patient's prognosis will be good no matter what she does. But if it's in a middle to late stage, the prognosis is usually negative. If someone comes in at a late stage in the disease, treatments generally won't work because the disease process is likely irreversible. I'm reluctant to say one way is better than another. But I do feel the current conventional system is shutting things down in patients and overriding their systems with chemical interventions. Homeopathy is different. We say, "Let's find the cause, and let's allow you and your body to self-correct." I see a lot of good results, but I can't predict with certainty.

What screening procedures do you recommend?
If you have five CT scans over a lifetime, I think it's almost guaranteed that you'll get cancer. Mammography has its place, but because of the

radiation, which is cumulative, it increases the risk of cancer. MRIs aren't benign, though we don't yet know how much damage they are causing. Ultrasound is the most benign of that group and has its place in identifying and tracking fibrocystic findings. In my opinion, thermography offers an effective screening tool for all women, but especially younger women who have denser breast tissue. It evaluates physiology and how the breasts function on a metabolic level, while mammography looks at structural changes. Since change occurs first on the level of physiology before it develops into a structural change, thermography is an excellent warning system to identify women in high-risk groups. It uses no radiation, no compression, and no contact — it just measures temperature that comes to the surface of the skin. It's not perfect, but when used in conjunction with structural tests when necessary, we get very good results. What I like about it is that it is highly predictive and can be used as an early warning system. Only one in ten biopsies leads to positive results. If we used thermography more frequently, we could reduce unnecessary biopsies substantially.

Breast cancer screening procedures

CT scan
Computerized tomography is a combined X-ray and computer procedure that exposes patients to high doses of radiation.

Mammogram
Mammography is an X-ray procedure that exposes patients to radiation that is one hundred times that of a chest X-ray. It does not pass through vital organs (such as the brain, heart, or lungs) and stays in the breasts, which are compressed during the procedure.

MRI
Magnetic resonance imaging uses magnets and radio waves, rather than radiation, to create images of "slices" of the body.

Thermogram
Thermography involves using an infrared camera to record temperature. The technique is a safe and non-invasive one based on the idea that the temperature of abnormal cells is higher than that of normal cells because of increased blood flow. Thermograms do not use ionizing radiation, which is used in CT scans and X-rays and can cause DNA damage.

Ultrasound
Ultrasound, or sonography, is a procedure that uses high-frequency sound waves that bounce off surfaces to create images.

What is your cure rate with breast cancer patients?

When someone comes in with a complex disease like cancer, I'm reluctant to give a prognosis. I'm very confident with certain conditions like migraines and irritable bowel syndrome, where I have a 70 to 90 percent success rate. But cancer is multifactorial, so it's hard to predict. The solution is to not get it. That's where I feel I'm most effective: prophylactically. Of the thousands of long-term patients I've worked with over the years, perhaps less than 2 percent get cancer. That's a lot better than your average statistic. No women in my practice who have been seeing me for two, three, four, or five years get breast cancer. The women in my practice who have breast cancer come to me with it. So I guess we are doing something right. It's holistic medicine, it's proactive, and it's prophylactic. That's the type of preventive medicine I'm happy with.

Holistic medicine
Holistic medicine considers physical, psychological, and social factors in order to improve a patient's condition.

CHAPTER 7

Dr. Ahmad Nasri,
Homeopath, Naturopath

Shortly after completing my own treatment, I met with Dr. Nasri. His unassuming clinic, located on the outskirts of Toronto, belied his devotion to the important work he has conducted with cancers at all stages over the last twenty years. Subsequent to completing a Bachelor of Science degree in Lebanon, Dr. Nasri received his medical and surgical training in the Dominican Republic, where he also worked as medical director of a holistic clinic that treated patients with late-stage cancers. There, he was introduced to the work of Dr. Rudy Falk, a Canadian oncologist and conventionally-trained surgeon who was doing pioneering work in the 1980s in Canada, integrating alternative treatments such as Poly-MVA into mainstream oncology. Dr. Nasri was impressed with the beneficial effects that treatments such as ozone autohemotherapy, dendritic cell vaccines and targeted low-dose chemotherapy had on these difficult-to-treat late-stage cancers. When Dr. Falk died, Dr. Nasri relocated to Toronto, where he trained as a homeopath and was in the process of adding naturopathic training to his list of accreditations at the time of this interview.

> Poly MVA is a mineral and vitamin complex that is administered intravenously and has antioxidant and detoxifying properties. It is regarded as safe with no side effects.

Ozone autohemotherapy is a 30 to 40 minute procedure where about 250 ml of blood drawn from the patient is exposed to ozone, then re-injected into the patient via an intravenous procedure. This oxygenates the blood and gives the patients energy.

Dendritic cell vaccines have been found in some cases to cause anti-tumour immune responses in various cancers.

Dr. Nasri, what do you think causes breast cancer?

Environmental toxicity, hormonal imbalance, unhealthy diet, poor weight management, and genetics are all causes. We used to blame genetics for many cancers, but now we are seeing young patients with breast cancer and no genetic loading. This is an environmental issue.

When should a woman with breast cancer come to you?

A woman with breast cancer should come to me as early as possible, but when a woman finds a lump, she usually goes to her GP [general medical practitioner] and is sent for a mammogram or ultrasound, and then a biopsy, and that's how things start (they then may proceed down a conventional medical path). After diagnosis, it is important that people become well informed about all treatment options, including alternative ones, before choosing a course of treatment.

What do you think about surgery?

I'd definitely recommend surgery. Generally, from a holistic approach, if you can get rid of the tumour and then do treatments, you have a better outcome. Surgery, even the biopsy, has the potential to cause the cancer cells to spread, but the pros of surgery outweigh the cons. Before deciding which treatment to pursue, however, I'd check a patient's tumour markers (CA 15-3 for breast cancer, CA 125 for ovarian cancer, and PSA for prostate cancers), which indicate how aggressive the cancer is. These tests give us baseline readings and help us to determine if the tumour is responding to the treatment that is chosen, whether that's conventional or complementary. For example, after surgery, the tumour markers will go down to almost a normal range because you have removed the tumour. If the patient has declined surgery, tumour markers will remain at a certain level as long as the immune system is functioning well enough to keep the cancer in check. I've seen the lesion remain stable for years in some of my patients who refuse surgery and other conventional interventions. However, increased stress can result in a sudden increase in size of the tumour and rapid deterioration of the patient's state. At any point before or after surgery, if the tumour markers are rising even with complementary therapy, this is a red flag and suggests that the lesions have spread. This might indicate the need for using conventional treatments like chemo adjunctively.

When a patient decides to proceed with surgery, the question of which surgery to do is also important. You don't need to rush to do a mastectomy when a lumpectomy might be sufficient.

What do you think about chemotherapy and radiation?

I'm not against treatments such as chemo and radiation, but we don't need to rush into chemo right away. Chemo does work in some cases, but research has shown that it may not provide full remission for stages III and IV on its own with the current conventional protocol. Because the collateral damage of chemo is terrible, the chances of surviving beyond five years may be better when chemo is not used right away in stage I or II. Additionally, we need to consider other treatments where possible because of this collateral damage. I usually tell my patients with early stage breast cancer that chemo is always there, but alternative treatments can work well with stage I patients. I'd usually recommend doing two to three months of alternative therapy first and then decide, depending how successful these interventions are.

In those cases where it's necessary — for instance, in stage III or IV, or if the alternative treatment alone hasn't arrested the cancer — you need to prepare the body to deal with the side effects of chemo by building up the immune system and balancing the organs with, for instance, diet and supplementation. This is where complementary treatment can be helpful. Unfortunately, many allopathic doctors tell patients not to take powerful antioxidants during chemo. They argue that they might interfere with the chemo action. Many patients are then frightened to take these, though they minimize collateral damage. To the contrary, research has shown a synergism between some chemo agents and alternative treatments, and in fact, alternative treatment can actually augment the beneficial effects of the chemo. If the blood counts are low and the patient is anaemic, this needs to be dealt with before chemo, as the chemo will further affect this. The liver may need detoxifying. Milk thistle and dandelion can help with this.

Moreover, in advance of deciding on a particular treatment, there are many more options now even before surgery. You have genetic tests, like the oncogene test, that help the oncologist determine which chemo the tumour is most sensitive to or whether chemo can be effective at all. There are low-dose chemotherapies that are better because they minimize side effects, and there is chronomodulated chemo, which is a chemo given at different times of the day to be more effective. However, chronomodulated chemo is used mainly in Germany, not here. There are many options, and the complementary and allopathic approaches diverge a lot around which choices to make. We in the complementary medicine community need to do more research and demonstrate the effectiveness of our interventions to doctors in the allopathic community.

Radiation may be even worse than chemo. You cause free radical damage and genetic mutation on the chromosomal level, which can lead to other cancers later. In order to prevent future side effects after radiation, I administer antioxidants such as vitamin C, glutathione (known as the body's most powerful antioxidant), and alpha lipoic acid (a synthetic version of lipoic acid that is an antioxidant vital to cellular energy production). These are free radical scavengers, which rid the body of free radicals. Under normal circumstances our bodies are programmed to employ antioxidants to do this work. However, with radiation, our body's immune system needs help. Mushroom and thymus extracts can be employed to help boost immune functioning. The liver should be checked through blood testing to ensure adequate detoxifying and that the natural killer cells are doing their work. These blood test results can help us monitor the present state of disease and future risks.

More specifically, what are the interventions you employ and which would you say are most important?
Unfortunately, we don't have the studies to say which interventions are better, so we use them in combination, and that gives us the best results. I've learned over my more than seventeen years doing this work that you can't just do one modality — the interventions work best synergistically. For example, with cancer you can't just focus on diet.

It's also important to have an individualized approach because every person's needs are different. In conventional treatments, professionals have a protocol that is the same for everybody, but I feel that's a mistake. We combine oral interventions — that is supplementation, which patients do at home — with intravenous treatments that patients have in the clinic two to three times weekly. The initial treatment phase comprises around twenty intravenous sessions, after which patients continue with maintenance therapy. These treatments include a mix of vitamins, minerals, and biological modulators that act on the cancer cells specifically by intervening in their energy production and causing them to die. Other substances, like homeopathics, are added to the mix to help support the immune system in getting rid of the cancer and to help specific organs that are affected, like liver, lymphatic system, and intestines.

Homeopathic remedies are administered to help with the side effects of chemotherapy, such as anemia, nausea, and vomiting. Oral supplementation with cancer-specific substances is taken on the days when patients are not receiving intravenous therapy. Hormonal imbalance is also always addressed during the treatment — for example, estrogen dominance in patients with hormone-sensitive tumours, like with some breast cancers. These patients have an over-production of estrogen, so we increase the progesterone and balance and inhibit estrogen receptors in susceptible organs like the breast and uterus through diet, and with supplements like indole-3-carbinol, DIM, and Vitex. Stress reduction is another pillar in an effective treatment, so we use reflexology, reiki, Neuro-Linguistic Programming and biofeedback to identify sources of stress and help the body decrease its effect on the immune system. Studies show that the immune system capacity (measured through IgA levels) is directly reduced during stress.[31]

> Neuro-Linguistic Programming attempts to improve certain psychological and medical conditions by changing a person's perception, thinking and behaviour.

How long should patients stay on your protocol?

Treatment plans are individualized and depend on the staging of each patient and the treatments patients have already done. On average, I would say patients have about three months of aggressive treatment, then maintenance for one year. After one year, if the patient is fine and well educated about how to manage on their own with their diet, supplementation, lifestyle and stress reduction, then they will be on maintenance treatments and monitored every three to six months. If we do testing and it shows a patient has a higher risk of developing cancer, they might need longer use of supplementation to decrease the risk. Tumour markers tested in the blood should be done every six months, for the first couple of years, then after that once a year. These tests are covered under OHIP [the universal health care plan in Ontario]. Doing this is a way of getting ahead of the game. Patients have had a wake-up call with the initial diagnosis, and they need to be vigilant for five to ten years. I've seen patients who have not been vigilant for whom it's come back with a vengeance. Breast cancer can spread to the liver, lungs, bones, and brain, so any sudden bone pain or increase in liver enzymes needs to be attended to.

---

31   Segerstrom, S. C., & Miller, G. E. (2004). Psychological Stress and the Human Immune System: A Meta-Analytic Study of 30 Years of Inquiry. *Psychological Bulletin, 130*(4), 601-630. https://doi.org/doi:10.1037/0033-2909.130.4.601

What are your suggestions for an anti-cancer diet?

There are a lot of studies that show that people shouldn't eat certain foods when they have cancer and other diseases.[32] People should be having an anti-inflammatory, hypo-allergenic diet. Generally, chemicals in food, such as preservatives, as well as dairy and eggs, are all allergenic substances. Without doing individual testing, I'd recommend a dairy-free, gluten-free diet with, for example, organic chicken, fish, no red meats, and lots of vegetables and fruit. But these are general guidelines, and I like to do individual testing to determine which foods the patient's immune system reacts to. For example, while they might assume that juicing with broccoli or asparagus is good, some patients' immune systems won't benefit from this. I use IgG (immunoglobulin G, an antibody) and IgA (immunoglobulin A, an antibody) tests to determine which foods nourish the patient's immune system.

However, I'm not an extremist with diet, and I don't think going on a strict diet is going to cure you. If a person eats a piece of cake, it won't cause the cancer to come back right away. Coffee and cake three times a week is not good, but I don't worry about an occasional coffee. I worry more about the chemicals in the coffee; for instance, in decaffeinated coffee. Coffee can actually be helpful for blood pressure. Of course, they shouldn't eat lots of pizza, and a gluten-free diet will decrease the potential for inflammation. I don't agree with a lot that has been said about acidifying foods. It's important to keep our PH balanced, but I believe the focus on this is exaggerated because we have a well-designed internal system that regulates the PH (acid and alkaline balance) in our bodies. Of course, we should not be eating only acidic foods. But the stress of worrying about diet may be worse than the diet itself. Moderation is important. Patients become scared to eat things, and I've seen many patients on cancer diets, such as

---

32 Block G., Patterson, B., & Subar, A. (1992). Fruit, vegetables and cancer prevention: A review of the epidemiological evidence. *Nutrition and Cancer, 18*(1), 1-29. https://doi.org/10.1080/01635589209514201

macrobiotic, doing terribly and losing muscle mass because they are not getting the correct nutrition. You never want that to happen in cancer patients, because if they lose muscle mass, they are susceptible to a recurrence.

What do you see as important measures to prevent recurrence?

A holistic approach that considers diet, supplementation, intravenous treatments, and stress reduction is very important. Most patients with breast cancer had huge stressful events before their diagnosis. The first year after treatment is an especially precarious time, particularly around the incision, and it's a perfect time and a crucial window in which to support the immune system and prevent any recurrence. But patients treated allopathically are often abandoned after treatment, with little follow-up other than mammograms unless there is a recurrence.

If a person has a recurrence, can you help them?

Once a patient has had a recurrence, it minimizes the success of what I can do, but it also depends on the staging of the recurrence and whether it's metastasized. With stage II and III I'm able to keep the cancer stable and sometimes reverse disease. Stage IV with metastasis is more difficult. I get a lot of stage IV patients who have done many chemotherapies, perhaps some experimental, that give them many side effects and may only give them an extra month of life. These patients usually come to me on lots of medications for pain, stool softeners for constipation, vomiting, and are unable to eat with loss of appetite. If the breast cancer has spread to the bones, we can decrease pain. If they are on morphine for pain and you decrease the morphine, they are less constipated. Once they are less constipated they can eat better and improve their nutrition. Their immune system functioning improves, and their muscle mass increases. Often we can help these patients with a much-improved quality of life for up to a year.

How do you deal with the skepticism of mainstream doctors?

You try and do what you think you should do. There are big egos on both sides. I trained traditionally as a surgeon as well as a homeopath, which helps, and I've also dealt with a lot of patients. I try to be moderate, not extremist, and research what's out there, not just use it because others are talking about it. I usually speak about integrative cancer treatments to medical doctors. They are interested if you show them what's working and why. I get calls from doctors whose wives get cancer, or they themselves, and they want to be treated alternatively. Because of the power of Big Pharma, we don't have enough research studies; however, an increasing number of clinical trials are being conducted that evaluate and prove the validity of complementary therapies. I believe these will ultimately convince skeptical minds.

It's a problem that some alternative therapists are claiming that certain therapies are miraculous without basing it on sound research. For example, you can't tell people that a certain supplement is guaranteed to cure an advanced cancer unless you have clinical evidence to back it up. We need to be honest and while remaining hopeful, not give cancer patients and their families unrealistic hope. I'm very clear with patients. I never promise what I can't deliver. If I see a patient who is terminal and likely to die in a couple of months, I'll be clear about what we can do. To do otherwise causes a lot of damage, both to the patient and to our reputation.

CHAPTER 8

Dr. Fred Hui, Integrative Physician

Dr. Hui's medical philosophy, which integrates Eastern and Western medicine, both complementary and allopathic, reflects his life experience. He grew up in Hong Kong and then immigrated to Canada, where he trained as a medical doctor in Toronto. He is now lecturing in the faculties of medicine at the University of Toronto and McMaster University in Hamilton. He has spent time with practitioners across the globe who have done fascinating things to cure cancer and who have had many successes. As Dr. Hui shared these stories with me, a sense of both excitement and dismay arose in me. I learned of amazing interventions that have had profound effects for some patients, but in some instances, have been shut down by, for instance, powerful lobbies such as the pharmaceutical industry. Nevertheless, I felt hopeful that if people could come together from disparate parts of the world and opposite ends of the professional spectrum, as Dr. Pettle writes in the foreword of this book, we could come up with a much-improved toolkit to treat this elusive disease.

Dr. Hui, what can one do to prevent breast cancer?
I believe there are two types of cancer: sexual organ cancers, such as breast, ovarian, and prostate, that are driven by hormone imbalance; and virus-based cancers, such as lung, pancreas, and colon. Regarding breast cancer, certain hormonal interventions can help to prevent the onset and recurrence. Progesterone is one hormone that I like

very much. The progesterone receptor in the adrenal glands serves as the "off" switch for the cancer activity. I concur with Dr. John Lee, who presents the utility of progesterone as a moderating factor (i.e., it keeps the hormones in balance) in breast cancer in his book *What Your Doctor May Not Tell You About Breast Cancer.* Excessive estrogen causes an overstimulation of estrogen sensitive tissues such as the brain, uterus lining, and breast glands, and early indications that this is occurring include heavy periods, premenstrual syndrome, and tender breasts. These symptoms of estrogen dominance suggest there is insufficient progesterone to balance the estrogen. Often, doctors who are presented with these symptoms in their clinical work neglect to address the chronic underlying imbalance, perhaps only removing the breast lump or the fibroid in the uterus. However, this is a short-term solution. The imbalance will continue to grow if dealt with in this way, causing some people to eventually end up with breast cancer. There is no known dietary way to increase progesterone; therefore, the only way to moderate this estrogen overload either in the breast or uterus is a dash of progesterone administered topically in the second half of the menstrual cycle. Progesterone is also used in conventional medicine to balance hormones with, for example, uterine cancer.

Dr. John Lee

Dr. Lee was a pioneer and expert in natural hormone replacement. His book *What Your Doctor May Not Tell You About Breast Cancer* highlights how women can help prevent breast cancer and recurrences by balancing estrogen and progesterone, while also being attentive to other breast cancer contributing factors such as diet, environment and stress. Dr. Lee was outspoken about his beliefs that many conventional cancer treatments were not working. He encouraged doctors to question the influence of the drug companies in their treatment choices and discuss and explore alternative interventions with colleagues and patients.[33]

33   Lee, J. R., Zava, D., & Hopkins, V. (2002). *What your doctor might not tell you about breast cancer: How hormone balance can help save your life.* New York, NY: Warner books.

How is estrogen metabolized?

Estrogen is metabolized into 2 hydroxyestrogen (good) or 4 or 16 hydroxyestrogen (both bad). Supplements like indol-3-carbinol and DIM, as well as cruciferous vegetables, such as brussel sprouts and broccoli, will aid in ensuring pathways go to the good estrogen (2 hydroxyestrogen). Some breast cancer patients need estrogen supplementation to ensure the hormones are balanced. I like to use topical bio-identical hormones such as BiEst, which is 80% estriol (the good guy) and 20% estradiol (the brain requires this to properly function). I also use transdermal estriol cream, a cream that is applied through the skin, as a preventative measure. There is controversy regarding foods such as soy that contain estrogen, but if you look at breast cancer in Japan and China, their incidence is lower despite heavy consumption of soy products such as tofu and miso. The explanation for this is that the estrogen found in these foods tends to be a weak form, and when it attaches to the estrogen receptors, it leaves no room for the bad estrogen to attach.

> Soy contains phytoestrogens which are plant based compounds that have a structure that is similar to estrogen. They are referred to as weak estrogens.

However, in patients with an estrogen-positive breast cancer, excess estrogen (that is, excess estrone or estradiol) will feed the cancer. This excess can occur in many ways. External sources like non-organic meat can deposit residues of hormones from the animal in our bodies. Post-menopausal women do not have ovaries that produce hormones; however, some estrogen is still produced by adrenal glands. I don't like using DHEA supplementation with estrogen-sensitive cancer patients because, from a biochemical point of view, DHEA is a precursor of estrogen, which can potentially cause a recurrence by feeding the growth of the hormone-sensitive cancer cells. This may happen because DHEA can produce extra testosterone, which can then be converted into estrogen (called aromatization, a process whereby the body converts testosterone into a female hormone). It is impossible to properly monitor DHEA supplementation, and by the time you discover a lump that might indicate it has caused a recurrence, it's too late. However, DHEA in patients who do not have cancer is preventative. It will rewind the internal clock, making the biological age younger and improving the immune functioning of the body, inducing health.

What about using melatonin in cancer prevention?

I love melatonin. Cancer is mostly age-related and melatonin is anti-aging ; therefore, I feel it contributes to cancer prevention. The body becomes depleted of melatonin as you age, so if you artificially wind the body clock backwards and the body thinks it's, say, only twenty years of age, the cancer won't germinate.[34] People could start using melatonin from middle age (their forties) as a prophylaxis. If they have had poor sleep from early in their lives, they were probably born with low melatonin levels and could usefully supplement with melatonin earlier in their life. Melatonin is great for all cancers because if you improve a person's sleep, you can strengthen their immune system, they can better fight off illness, and there are no contraindications with cancer patients. My instructions to patients are to take one 3-milligram tab the first night, two tabs (6 milligrams) the second night, three tabs (9 milligrams) the third night and so on up to 20 milligrams per night. In order for melatonin to be effective, you must sleep in a dark room, so use an eye cover if necessary. The dosage is correct if you wake up in a dark room and you want to sleep more and if you feel rested when you awaken in the morning. Unlike sleeping pills, its effects don't linger in the day. Melatonin is cheap and easily

---

34   Hill, S. M., Cheng, C., Yuan, L., Mao, L., Jockers, R., Dauchy, B., & Blask, D. E. (2013). Age-related decline in melatonin and its MT1 receptor are associated with decreased sensitivity to melatonin and enhanced mammary tumor growth. *Current Aging Science,* 6(1), 125-133. Retrieved from https://www.ncbi.nlm.nih.gov/pubmed/23895529

available. Melatonin levels cans be checked with urine and saliva tests performed in the US.

I spent some time in Italy with Dr. Luigi Di Bella, a physician and physiology professor, who convinced me of the beneficial effects of melatonin with cancer patients.[35] He believed that the malignant tumour can co-exist peacefully with the body, and while maybe you won't cure cancer patients, you can maintain them and they can still live a good quality of life, even with the cancer. Melatonin was an important part of his treatment, and he put every cancer patient on 20 milligrams of melatonin a day because he believed rewinding the body clock would enable the body to better fight off infections. [His therapy included a drug cocktail containing melatonin, retinoids, vitamins E, D3 and C, bromocriptine, and somatostatin; and low-dose cyclophosphamide, a chemo drug. He believed this cocktail offered low toxicity, higher rates of survival and a better quality of life for all stages and kinds of cancer when compared with chemotherapy.[36]]

Dr. Di Bella's cancer treatment was controversial. Despite this, an editorial in the *British Medical Journal* in 1999 suggested that multicentre clinical trials conducted by Italian researchers to examine the efficacy of Di Bella's treatments were poorly designed. The author said that because there were no control groups for comparison, the utility or otherwise of Di Bella's treatment could not be definitively proven.[37] Other studies have reported benefits of Di Bella's protocol.

35 Di Bella, G. (2013). Anti-cancer effects: Review. *International Journal of Molecular Science, 14*(2), 2410-2430. https://doi.org/10.3390/ijms14022410

36 Di Bella, G. (2010). The Di Bella method (DBM). *Neuro Endocrinology Letters, 31*(Suppl. 1), 1-42. Retrieved from https://www.ncbi.nlm.nih.gov/pubmed/20881933

37 Mullner, M. (1999). Di Bella's therapy: The last word? The evidence would be stronger if the researchers had randomized their studies. *British Medical Journal, 318*(7178), 208-209. Retrieved from https://www.ncbi.nlm.nih.gov/pmc/articles/PMC1114705/

For instance, a study conducted in 2001 reported that Di Bella's treatment protocol offered benefits to 70% of those patients studied who had advanced stage non-Hodgkin lymphoma.[38]

What are some other useful interventions for hormonally driven cancers?

I feel arimidex and tamoxifen are useful in some patients with breast cancer because both of them suppress the body's production of hormones. Arimidex blocks the conversion of male hormones (testosterone) to female hormones (estrogen), and tamoxifen puts a woman into artificial menopause. Tamoxifen and arimidex are useful in managing excess estrogen, but they have side effects. Tamoxifen can cause depression, hot flashes, and aging skin, and it may affect your immune system because it ages you. But if a patient is at high risk for breast cancer due to family history or for other reasons, I'd say take tamoxifen or aromatase inhibitors. This way, even patients with metastasis may live on and die of something else.

I like to use vitamin C intravenously for all cancer patients. I follow the protocol developed by Dr. Hugh Riordan, who believed that this intervention could limit the growth of the cancer.[39] Vitamin C in high doses metabolizes into hydrogen peroxide. Since cancer cells, unlike regular cells, don't have the catalase enzyme to break down the hydrogen peroxide, the intravenous vitamin C acts like a smart bomb- killing cancer cells.

---

38 Todisco, M., Casaccio, P., & Rossi, N. (2001). Cyclophosphamide plus somatostatin, bromocriptine, retinoids, melatonin and ACTH in the treatment of low-grade non-Hodgkin's lymphomas at advanced stage: Results of a phase II trial. *Cancer Biotherapy and Radiopharmaceuticals, 2,* 171-177. https://doi.org/10.1089/108497801300189263

39 Padayatty, S. J., Riordan, H. D., Hewitt, S. M., Katz, A., Hoffer, L. J., & Levine, M. (2006). Intravenously administered vitamin C as cancer therapy: Three cases. *Canadian Medical Association Journal, 174*(7), 937-942. https://doi.org/10.1503/cmaj.050346

Essiac tea is another potentially helpful product. I have had good feedback from patients about this. It is available and cheap, and you just need to follow the instructions for using it. It can be purchased online or in some health food stores.

There are other amazing treatments out there. Ukrain is one such drug. My patients had this affordable medication shipped to them, then they brought it to me and I administered it intravenously to them. I thought I had become a miracle doctor with this tool in my hand, because in almost forty years of practice, I've never seen results like this with anything else. I've recommended it to so many patients, and they've had obvious and dramatic recoveries from cancer without the side effects. Ukrain eventually dries the cancer up. I have treated patients with pancreatic cancer with Ukrain, and to date, they have survived more than five years. If you can treat pancreatic cancer, you can treat anything.

Ukrain

Ukrain is a drug derived from the great celandine flower, a plant that has been well known in herbal medicine for more than three thousand years. Studies conducted with Ukrain alone or in combination with chemo drugs claim that Ukrain is the only anti-cancer drug that accumulates immediately after administration in the cancer cells, triggering the death of the cancer cells. Unlike most other drugs, supporters claim it dries up the malignant cells, while leaving healthy cells intact and also boosts the immune system. A review of data of clinical trials of UKRAIN up to 2014 concluded that this drug had potential as an anti-cancer drug, but that large scale studies are required to confirm its effect.[40,41,42]

Dr. Wassil Nowicky, a Ukrainian chemist, who studied in Austria and eventually became a citizen there, developed Ukrain into a form that could be administered intravenously to patients with cancer.

There is a herbal based formula that is used in Asia to treat the flu, called Xiao Chai Hu Tang Wan, or Minor Bupleurum Decoction. There is a herbalist by the name of Dr. Ma Hong Chau in Hong Kong who uses this product with minor modifications to treat cancer patients. Its use is based on the virus theory of cancer, which makes sense to me. I have seen patients with metastatic breast cancer, which had spread to the bone, alive and well four years after commencing a course of this herbal treatment. This suggests that, despite being a treatment for viral cancers, it seems also to work with some sexual hormone cancers like breast cancer. My hypothesis is that with sexual hormone cancers, a virus caused the cancer and some hormones feed it. The theory behind this herbal intervention is that a virus got into the cellular system screwing it up, but it remains resistant to attack by the immune system. The virus, which is a strand of DNA, imbeds itself in the nucleus of the host cells, living intracellularly and attacking the DNA of other cells, and then uses the body energy to facilitate

---

40   Ernst, E., & Schmidt, K. (2005). Ukrain – A new cancer cure? A systematic review of randomised clinical trials. *BMC Cancer, 5*(69). https://doi.org/10.1186/1471-2407-5-69

41   Uglyanitsa, K. N., Nefyodov, L. I., Doroshenko, Y. M., Nowicky, J. W., Volchek, I. V., Brzosko, W. J., & Hodysh, Y. J. (2000). Ukrain: a novel antitumor drug. *Drugs under Experimental and Clinical Research, 26*(5-6), 341-356. Retrieved from https://www.ncbi.nlm.nih.gov/pubmed/11345050/?ncbi_mmode=std

42   Memorial Sloan Kettering Cancer Center. (2014, November 11). *About herbs, botanicals, and other products.* Retrieved from https://www.mskcc.org/cancer-care/diagnosis-treatment/symptom-management/integrative-medicine/herbs

reproduction of the cancer cells. The herbal medicine exposes the virus that caused the cancer (proliferation of abnormal, malignant cells) so that the body's immune system can see it, and attack and kill it. When this battle is over between the cells, the patient is cured. The patients are prescribed an herbal mix that is tailored to their particular situation and is constantly adjusted throughout the course of their treatment according to their condition.

I learned about this treatment from an old medical school friend from Hong Kong. He got esophageal cancer, had surgery, refused chemo and radiation, and subsequently consulted the herbalist. Since using this treatment, he has not had any recurrence. He told me about some of the recoveries he witnessed and suggested I visit. I spent three days in this clinic talking to some of the patients in the waiting room, and I witnessed his results first hand, like the jaundiced patient with advanced liver cancer whose liver indexes after three years are normal, with no evidence of the cancer. If any doctor can turn around one in ten cancers, he should be happy, but I think this doctor's success is much higher based on my contact with survivors who come back to him. The treatment is cheap and available, so people don't think it's a powerful treatment, but he treats end-stage cancer with good results. This treatment is not available here in Canada, but there is a Chinese herbalist in New Mexico who practices this method. If I discovered I had cancer tomorrow, I would go to Hong Kong and have this treatment.

What do you think about surgery, radiation, and chemotherapy?

I feel surgery is definitely useful in ridding the body of cancer. Radiation is localized; it's like giving the body sunburn, and can still offer the chance of a cure. But chemo is a different matter — I'm very hesitant to use it. I believe only a few cancers respond to chemo; for example, childhood leukemia, testicular cancer, and lymphoma, but even with lymphoma I believe in the virus theory, which precludes the use of chemo. When conventional treatments such as chemo or radiation are used, they act like an atomic bomb blasting the site of the mass. But this radical approach not only kills the lymphocytes that were in effect the "good guys" acting as a kind of police force, trying to contain the virus, but it also burns the earth around, which contained healthy cells. If you are lucky enough to kill only the virus, the patient may recover, but too often the police and healthy cells are wiped out and the patient dies from the devastation wreaked by the treatment.

Do you think the body can recover after chemo?

Yes, I believe the body can recover and rebuild given the right interventions. When people come to me in a terrible physical state after a conventional treatment, I look at every aspect of their functioning. With my protocol, which is based on Dr. Jacob Teitelbaum's book *From Fatigued to Fantastic,* I examine, for instance, sleep, hormones, infections, and nutrition. As I mentioned earlier, I immediately try and improve their sleep by getting them on 20 milligrams of melatonin. I also look at, amongst other things, the state of their hormones (for example, the adrenals), their thyroid functioning, infections like fungal or mycoplasma that may have invaded their immune system while it was depressed by the disease and further by the treatments, and finally their nutritional status, including, for example, iron content and vitamin D, which are important in fighting infections. The adrenals are a stabilizing gland against things like jet lag, weather change and temperature regulation, allergies, low blood sugar and low blood pressure. Most people who have had chemo present with adrenals that are depleted. If you are still tired after you wake up and have low blood pressure, low blood sugar, cold hands and feet, and frequent urination, the adrenal functioning is too low. In Chinese medicine, this is called adrenal deficiency syndrome. (See my website, www. drhui.com, on chronic adrenal fatigue syndrome).

Naturopaths tend to focus on detoxifying the liver by, for example, eating more vegetables and cutting out coffee, but it's more complicated than that because when people are deficient, their bodies need nourishment. Vegan diets do not adequately nourish the body for people with low adrenals because the body gets too cold and you become weak. Something like coffee may be good for some people in moderation because it bumps up the functioning of the adrenals if they are low. When it comes to diet, it's not one-size-fits-all, but needs to be individualized based on adrenal functioning, kidney functioning, and so on.

CHAPTER 9

Dr. Charles Hayter, Radiation Oncologist

By a stroke of good fortune, I stumbled upon *Radical,* a play written by Dr. Charles Hayter, while attending the Toronto Fringe Festival in the summer of 2014. The play is the story of Vera Peters, a radiation oncologist at Princess Margaret Hospital in Toronto in the seventies, who spearheaded a revolution against the mass application of radical mastectomies. At that time, such mastectomies were being performed on almost all women with breast cancer, no matter what their age or stage of breast cancer. Dr. Peters gathered data on eight thousand women to support her hypothesis that radical mastectomies were not always warranted for a good treatment outcome.[43] She also believed that surgery alone could cure women with small breast cancers of less than two centimetres. Dr. Peters believed that women should have a voice in their treatment choices. Charles Hayter, also a radiation oncologist and medical historian, brought this important story to our attention again through his play, highlighting the pioneering efforts of one woman in her fight against a conservative medical system. He has reminded us that, as in the case of Vera Peters, a belief in a

---

43 Cowan, D. H. (2010). Vera Peters and the conservative management of early-stage breast cancer. *Current Oncology, 17*(2), 50-54. Retrieved from https://www.ncbi.nlm.nih.gov/pmc/articles/PMC2854638/

medical practice that is outside of the mainstream of the time can initiate a revolution that ultimately changes the course of treatment in medicine. In this case, Vera Peters' research and beliefs ultimately had a profound impact in the treatment of breast cancer. I am very grateful for Dr. Hayter's generosity in sharing this inspiring story and his thoughts with me during this interview.

Vera Peters

Vera Peters was born in 1911 in a suburb of Toronto and later attended the University of Toronto, where she pursued a medical degree after studies in math and physics. While in medical school, and as a consequence of her mother's illness with breast cancer, she became acquainted with the Head of Radiotherapy at Toronto General Hospital, Dr. Gordon Richards, an acquaintance who was instrumental in her decision later to study radiation oncology. Vera Peters was very disturbed by both the disfigurement caused by mastectomy and the emotional impact of this procedure on women. In 1975, she presented ground breaking research that showed that women who were treated with lumpectomy and radiation for early stage breast cancer had the same rate of cure as women who had undergone mastectomy. Though these findings were met with resistance from the surgical lobby, they ultimately contributed to the replacement of this radical practice in many cases with lumpectomy. While she was not the first person to suggest alternatives to radical mastectomy in some patients, she was the first to carry out "appropriate controlled studies."[44]

---

44   Hayter, C. (2016). Vera Peters and the fight against breast cancer, *Heritage Matters, 14*(1), 11-12. Retrieved from https://www.heritagetrust.on.ca/en/pages/publications/ heritage-matters-magazine/heritage-matters-archives

What does your play suggest about breast cancer care and patient experience?

There's an adage in writing that you write about what you know, and what you are drawn to, and though Vera Peters was a woman, and people question a play about a woman written by a man, the ideas that she espoused are what I'm drawn to as a physician. I was attracted to medicine by its human side, the interaction with people. However, when I got into medical school, I saw a lot of things that weren't human, such as patients being ignored, the patriarchal system with trainees. Vera Peters had similar concerns as I did. She was a radiation oncologist, but she was more concerned with the impact on people and the need to respect their particular wishes and values. The play isn't really about lumpectomy or mastectomy; it's about something that is close to my heart, about giving patients a voice in treatment choices. If Vera Peters were sitting in the room, she'd say the same. Here was a woman in the sixties and seventies struggling to have her ideas accepted in a male-dominated medical system, to get male surgeons to recognize the suffering they were causing women. Hard as she tried, she wasn't able to change the practice herself, but she planted the seeds of change, while the surgeons eventually took up the fight and changed the practice.

What do you think are the causes of breast cancer?

Breast cancer was part of my practice until six or seven years ago, but now I do a lot of male genitourinary cancers, below the waist, including prostate and testicular, and gastrointestinal cancers such as rectal, stomach, and bladder. We doctors are mostly site-specific because there's so much information coming out with all cancers that no one person can keep up. With respect to cancer, people often ask "What caused my cancer?" but we don't really know what causes most cancers. There are probably a host of things that come together, such as genetic disposition, environment, diet, and chemicals. For instance, sun exposure causes skin cancer, and we know that breast cancer is partly related to diet, partly environmental, and partly familial.

How long do you think it will take to sort out the genesis of cancer?

All cancers have a genetic component; that is, something in the genes of cells turns on cell division. We all make cancers all the time, but our immune system recognizes them and deals with these abnormal cells. But we don't yet know which switch turns on the genes that cause the replication and why the immune system, which should be surveying things and killing bad cells, isn't doing its job. Solving this issue is very difficult because the biochemical pathways, the on/off triggers of cancer, make it complex. Moreover, I don't think we'll find there is a single factor that causes cancers. Cancer is about two thousand different diseases, and some cancers like prostate cancer have many subtypes. It's possible each kind has its own cause or combination of causes, which also makes finding a cure difficult. Sometimes a discovery makes the genesis more mystifying because the more we understand, the less we understand. When I was in medical school in Kingston in the eighties, a group of researchers found that killer cells scavenged cancer cells. At that time, everyone thought this was a huge breakthrough, but it just led to more questions. On the other hand, there have been giant breakthroughs in medical treatment in the last century or more. For example, in 1895 the discovery of X-rays was almost completely accidental and allowed us to look inside a living body. Maybe one hundred or two hundred years from now, they'll do gene therapy for certain cancers where you can re-program the cells and stop them from dividing, but we're currently far from that.

Given that we don't know specifically what causes cancer, are there things people can do to prevent it?

Toxins from cigarette smoke go everywhere in the body and can contribute to bladder cancer, though most people don't realize this. Diet is also a major factor. Asian people get upper GI tract cancer (esophageal and stomach cancer), but when they move to the Western world, their offspring get colon cancer and other lower GI tract cancers. That suggests that our fat-laden diet contributes to this. But since nothing is proven about the genesis of most cancers, prevention is difficult.

Given that the genesis of most cancers, including breast, remains unproven, and it's uncertain how much current conventional interventions actually get to the root of the disease, do you feel it is a contradiction that conventional doctors are such strong proponents of conventional and often debilitating interventions, such as surgery, chemotherapy, and radiation?

For a lot of disease, we've found effective treatments only because the cause is beyond doubt. For example, one hundred years ago, diphtheria decimated the child population in cities. Suddenly it was discovered to be a bacterial infection, and now it's nearly wiped out. The same with syphilis. Since there was no treatment, people used to go insane because it went to the brain. Now it has been eradicated. But with cancer, we lag far behind these discoveries. A cubic centimetre of cancer has one billion cells in it already, and each has the potential to break off and spread. It's much harder to get to the root cause of cancer, and surgery, radiation, and chemotherapy are all crude treatments. With surgery, we know that as the cancer gets bigger, the chances of getting metastases are greater, so if you find the cancer early enough, when the tumour is still small, the person may be cured with surgery alone. But some cancers are hard to find early on. With skin cancers, you notice it quickly because it's external and you can remove it before it spreads. But with respect to lung cancer, lungs are filled with empty space, so something can grow there for a long time before a person starts getting symptoms like a cough and shortness of breath. By the time you operate, the cancer is often so big that few people are cured. Radiation and chemo are crude. They kill cancer cells that are dividing, but they are not directed at the underlying cause, which is probably related to the genetics of the cell.

Do you think that a woman with an early stage breast cancer can be cured just with surgery?

We know there are women who are cured with just surgery. In fact, towards the end of her life, Vera Peters wrote that women with small breast cancers less than two centimetres in size could be cured without radiation as long as the malignant tumour had been completely removed. However, if a woman chooses not to have the tumour removed, she's taking a risk that the cancer might get bigger and metastasize.

But it seems to me there are few MDs who would recommend foregoing radiation with most cancers.
It's all about risks. A woman could have no conventional treatment for breast cancer and there could be a certain risk, or she could have a lumpectomy and that would involve other risks. The big studies published in the eighties followed Vera Peters' thinking, where women were allocated to three arms: mastectomy, lumpectomy, and lumpectomy plus radiation. The studies found that women who had only a lumpectomy had a 30 percent chance of cancer coming back in the breast, but with radiation and lumpectomy, it was less than 10 percent. I used to give women these stats and let them choose. The stats show that the risks happen in 5 percent of patients who get radiation treatments. Elderly women over seventy are often offered just surgery. Women with early stage breast cancer nowadays buy a standard package of radiation and surgery, which is based on these studies from the eighties, in which women who had surgery and radiation had a much lower recurrence rate. I don't see it as black and white, or conventional versus alternative treatment. A woman is taking a risk no matter what she chooses.

What about the collateral damage?
There is no medical treatment that doesn't cause some collateral damage or some side effects. You need to look at the risk/benefit ratio; that is, the risk of collateral damage versus the risk of cancer coming back. For example, with radiation, we have tables of threshold doses for different organs in the body, based on 5 percent of people getting damage in five years. In the eighties, when I trained, everyone thought heart muscles were radiation-resistant; then a big study came out in the nineties that really changed practice. It looked at women with left-sided breast cancer (the side of their heart) who had radiation

and found that they had a higher risk of heart disease. Now, before treatment starts, they calculate how much dosage can be administered while still shielding the heart. Consequently, fewer women get that side effect. When we give people radiation, they have to sign consent to acknowledge that they have been told about the side effects. With respect to chemotherapy drugs, Adriamycin can cause heart damage.

Do you have any thoughts about how current treatments can be improved?

Medicine is always looking for new ways of treating and curing people with fewer side effects and less collateral damage. In the field of radiation, we're always thinking about whether radiation is appropriate in a particular situation. For example, in the last fifteen years, evidence has emerged that indicates that you don't need to treat certain prostate cancers with radiation.

Low-grade prostate cancers that are picked up on PSA [prostate-specific antigens] tests, the male equivalent of mammography testing, may not need irradiating. When I see men with low-grade cancers, I give them the option of waiting and watching it. For some men, surgery is sufficient, for others radiation is used if the cancer is bigger. When I was training, radiation was used in a lot of childhood cancers, but now it's mostly chemo that is used. This is because children's bodies are growing and changing and there is a risk that the radiation may cause another cancer. We are always looking at ways to be more specific with the patients we treat.

What do you feel about patients following a less conventional course of treatment?

Patients often ask me if I mind if they try this or that approach, and I'll say I don't mind because it's your body. I don't tell patients what to do; my job is to give patients the information they need to make their own decision. I advise them to not get involved in things if the provider is unable to advise them of any side effects or if the treatment will deplete their bank account. All conventional approaches have side effects, but often with non-conventional approaches, the allure is that they claim to have no side effects. But as time goes on, they are also found to have side effects. Nothing works 100 percent, and everything has some side effects. And everybody is moving in the same direction: to find something that cures people with no side effects. Moreover, the conventional path is based on scientific evidence; that is, if you do this to somebody with this kind of cancer, you'll have this chance of cure. There aren't many non-conventional therapies that have been as rigorously tested as conventional therapies in clinical trials, though they may promise a cure. Therefore, when someone offers a cure with a non-conventional approach, we need to be sure there are scientific grounds for that statement.

I'm a historian of medicine, and the history of medicine tells us that the majority of conventional treatments nowadays came to us from non-conventional medicine; therefore, I feel the distinction between conventional and non-conventional healing approaches is very artificial. For example, there was a doctor in the eighteenth century who accidentally discovered that a weed known as digitalis, or purple foxglove, could be ground up and administered to patients with heart failure and they would get better. Marie Curie discovered radium in rocks, as a naturally occurring substance in the earth, and we now use radium routinely. Radiation has been used to treat people with cancer since 1900. When it started, the medical profession looked at it askance. In the thirties and forties, it was shown to work and it then became part of mainstream medicine. Acupuncture is another example of an intervention that was regarded as hocus-pocus twenty-five years ago by mainstream medicine. Now family doctors practise it, and little by little it's infiltrated mainstream medicine. I have no problem working with alternative professionals who want to work with us. When I was a student in Kingston, I was lucky to have been able to use the expertise of a licensed naturopath who came to the clinic weekly to help patients with side effects. But so much of the time, alternative practitioners feel antagonism towards conventional practitioners and they don't want to work with us. Additionally, as I mentioned earlier, the impact of their interventions on patients hasn't been studied so much.

If you got cancer, would you follow a conventional course of treatment?
Of course. Everyone who gets cancer wants to get cured, and though I understand the collateral damage of various interventions, I'd be willing to take a risk on this in the service of being cured. If someone came at me with an alternative approach and data, I'd consider it, but I wouldn't ignore a conventional approach. I'd consider integrating them. But if I got prostate cancer tomorrow, I wouldn't exchange a conventional approach for alternative approach because I see a lot of men whose PSAs return to normal after radiation, and they are cured. But I'd certainly look at doing whatever I could do to feel better. Vera Peters wrote a piece about what she would do if she got breast cancer, and she said she would have all the regular tests, have the tumour removed, and be checked every two months.

If you were to plant the seeds for change, what would they be?
There aren't as many big changes now in oncology as there were thirty or forty years ago. Looking at genetics and targeting bad genes directly is where breakthroughs are now. When I was a medical student at Queen's University twenty-five years ago, one of the doctors there said radiation would be outmoded in ten years because it wasn't a specific enough treatment for cancer and didn't target the underlying cause. He felt that it would be replaced by gene therapy, which is more targeted and, therefore, he saw it as a magic bullet. Now, thirty years later, we're still using radiation. There must be some evidence that things in left field will work. I don't believe in that distinction between the two camps, conventional and non-conventional; however, people are more educated now and they don't accept things without scientific evidence.

CHAPTER 10

Dr. Shailendra Verma,
Medical Oncologist

Dr. Verma is a medical oncologist at the Ottawa Hospital Cancer Centre. During his career, which has spanned thirty years, he has been involved in many research projects and clinical trials that have related to his work with patients with breast cancer, melanoma, and sarcoma. His commitment to his work has extended to his involvement in regulatory process, educational programs, and advocacy.

Dr. Verma's devotion to the well-being of cancer patients was very apparent to me as he so generously gave up some of his precious time to share his ideas on cancer treatment now and in the future. I was struck by the reassuring and soothing quality of his manner as I conducted the interview, a factor that I'm sure contributes to the loyalty and well-being of his cancer patients.

Dr. Verma, what do you think causes breast cancer?
There has never been a single smoking gun that points to the cause of breast cancer, such as smoking is to head and neck cancer, but the biggest risk is likely aging. As a woman goes through each menstrual cycle in typical normal physiology, there is a normal proliferation of cells in the breast, and there is more opportunity for her to produce an abnormal cell. Therefore, the more menstrual cycles a woman goes through in a lifetime, as is the case with women who have early

menarche or late menopause, the greater the chance that she could have a defect in the cells. Hence it has been observed that pregnancy serves as a protective factor against breast cancer, because there's a period of time when menses have ceased and the breast is tranquil because there are no huge fluctuations in the hormone levels and the hormones are uniquely anti-cancer. [There is an excess of estriol and progesterone at this time, which are protective.]

Excess estrogen and insulin have been identified as causative factors in breast cancer and play a role in proliferative stress. Excess weight, smoking, and alcohol consumption are all drivers of insulin and estrogen overload and are powerful growth factors for breast cancer. In post-menopausal women who take estrogen supplements for menopausal symptoms, there is additive long-term estrogen exposure that has been shown to increase breast cancer risk, if used for more than five years. Environmental factors — for example, chemicals like plastics, phthalates, and hydrofluorocarbons — have also been viewed by some as contributing factors to breast cancer, but their causal role has not been ascertained to date, and I believe they play a small role.

What are preventative things we can do if normal aging is a risk factor?

Epidemiological studies have shown that exercise and maintaining a healthy weight can reduce the risk of breast cancer.[45] Additionally, we could be examining the possibility of early pregnancy or even pseudo-pregnancy to reduce the proliferative stress on the breast in young women. This has never been tested in a trial but remains a theoretical possibility. For women at high risk, anti-estrogens like tamoxifen or aromatase inhibitors (in post-menopausal women) have been demonstrated to reduce the risk of developing breast cancer.[46]

---

45   Nelson, N. J. (2012). Studies on how lifestyle factors may affect breast cancer risk and recurrence. *Journal of the National Cancer Institute, 104*(8), 574-576. https://doi.org/10.1093/jnci/djs213

46   Kennecke, H. F., Ellard, S., O'Reilly, S., & Gelmon, K. A. (2006). New guidelines for treatment of early hormone positive breast cancer

What are your thoughts about current treatments?

Cancer is a sophisticated and complex illness that has many differing biologies in different individuals. There is agreement that removal of the primary tumour, if it has not already obviously spread, is the first step towards cure in many patients. However, at the same time, surgeons don't want to produce terrible problems for patients, like lymphedema and arm dysfunction, so they are continually looking for routes to do less. For example, if they don't need to take out the axillary nodes, they won't. Rather, they may simply sample them through sentinel node biopsies to provide the prognostic information and guidance regarding the need for any additional therapy. Consequently, the collateral damage of surgery has improved dramatically.

> Sentinel node biopsy is a procedure which involves removing the first, or first few lymph nodes in the armpit, that is the node or nodes that are closest to the breast. They are then examined to determine if cancer cells are present and have spread to the lymphatic system. This procedure is usually done while the patient is undergoing the initial surgery for the breast cancer.

There are plenty of women out there who refuse chemotherapy and radiation and, rather consult a naturopath, or use natural or herbal remedies. But if they have high-risk features, such as an aggressive primary or nodal involvement, my own experience is that most will relapse. In my practice, I've rarely seen a woman who has refused surgery of her primary breast cancer who has not subsequently progressed and then has required more extensive surgery. There are clearly exceptions to this, but they are rare and we do not fully understand why this is the case. It is difficult to study such women and the multiple alternative therapies they undertake and, hence, difficult to

---

with tamoxifen and aromatase inhibitors. *British Columbia Medical Journal, 48*(3), 121-126. Retrieved from https://www.bcmj.org/articles/new-guidelines-treatment-early-hormone-positive-breast-cancer-tamoxifen-and-aromatase

draw any reliable conclusions regarding the benefits or risks of such therapies. It would be great if the mainstream scientific community could develop collaborations to help educate and inform patients more reliably.

What do you think about tamoxifen, given the side effects?
I'm one of the world's greatest fans of tamoxifen. The more I've looked at this medicine, the more I've come to respect its impact on women with an estrogen-driven breast cancer (estrogen-receptor-positive). It has reduced mortality in this population, and while it definitely has risks and side effects, the risks pale in comparison to the benefits. Of one thousand women, three hundred who take this drug will not have a recurrence.[47]

The side effects of tamoxifen (hot flashes, vaginal discharge, and the extremely rare side effect of endometrial cancer or thrombosis) seem more manageable then those of other anti-estrogens, such as aromatase inhibitors, which seem to provoke muscle aches, risk of osteoporosis, and joint pain. A woman who has had breast cancer is looking through the door of her mortality, and she knows that certain aspects of her breast cancer can lead to a recurrence, metastasis, or even death. While recurrence doesn't necessarily lead to death, the stakes are higher when a woman with breast cancer has a relapse, and taking anti-estrogens, even with their side effects, is generally more acceptable. However, the intention of adjuvant therapy is to avoid a relapse in the first place, and anti-estrogens are often indicated for five to ten years. Getting a woman through such a long time frame takes patience and compassion.

47 Radmacher, M. D., & Simon, R. (2000) Estimation of tamoxifen's efficacy for preventing the formation and growth of breast tumours. *Journal of National Cancer Institute, 92*(1), 48-53. https://doi.org/10.1093/jnci/92.1.48

What do you think about the utility of alternative practitioners with this disease?

In my opinion, the best trained alternative practitioners are naturopaths, but even talented naturopaths are uncertain as to whether interventions such as diet or antioxidants will prevent a recurrence of cancer. I'm not biased against such interventions, but they need to be supported by good data that has also been subjected to the same microscope on safety as conventional medicine. Conventional medicine is overseen by many authorities: professional societies and guidelines groups, provincial and federal regulators, hospital and regional quality watchdogs, etc. Above all, we have to uphold the expectation that we provide patients with up-to-date information and therapies that have been proven to improve a variety of outcomes, such as mortality and quality of life.

In my opinion, these safety measures or standards do not exist with many practitioners of non-conventional therapies because of lack of regulation and adjudication. While desirable, this can be difficult to achieve, as some non-conventional practitioners — like, for example, some of those who practice reiki — suggest that their interventions don't require the same conventional research measures because they believe that the curative factor in part is a belief in the interventions. I don't feel this is adequate; however, I do think there's been a generational shift in this regard, at least amongst naturopaths. I've come across more naturopaths in the last five years who are interested in doing research than I have in the last twenty. At the Integrative Cancer Centre in Ottawa, there have been laudable efforts to improve dialogue and more collaboration between conventional and complementary practitioners. I strive to ensure that patients get advice from well-trained professionals who are trustworthy and have data to back up their advice. Both sides should be open about what they can offer the patient, rather than engaging in competition with the other side. This way, patients can make a choice about treatments that is founded in research, whether it's conventional or alternative. Patients are caught in a vortex of conflicting information and have to make choices with inadequate information. They come to us and say the oncologist said this and the naturopaths that. This tension for the patients causes stress and has to stop.

What role do you think patients themselves should have in managing their health?

I think one of the great tragedies of cancer is that patients get caught up in the system and become so dependent on it that they experience a lack of self-efficacy. I'm not a fan of Big Pharma, and while it is critically important for many aspects of health care, we need to move away from the model of "a drug for every ailment" and try and help patients achieve more of a self-care stance where they are less dependent on drugs. I think that programs that offer complementary health care provide patients with tools such as diet, stress reduction, and exercise. All of these supply the energy the body needs to heal and empower the individual.

CHAPTER 11

Biological Dentistry

Biological dentistry involves minimizing the use of toxic chemicals in the mouth and safely removing amalgam fillings. I was made aware of its importance by my naturopath, Sat Dharam Kaur, who is convinced that toxic chemicals employed in dental practices contribute to illness. The more research I did, the more I concurred with her about the urgency of attending to any toxic substances in my mouth. Removing my amalgam fillings to deal with mercury off-gassing seemed a good place to start. The following information comes from discussions I have had with several biological dentists.

The Connection between Oral Health and Overall Health

People are often surprised to hear that whatever you put in your mouth gets into your body, even if you don't swallow it. The most damaging way a poison enters your body is straight into your blood stream via the mouth, rather than ingesting it. When we have a case of food poisoning and become very ill, the body's natural defence and way of ridding itself of the poison it has ingested is to vomit or excrete it via the bowels. However, dental materials used in the mouth get into the body through mucosal membranes or blood or by being inhaled directly into the lungs, bypassing the gastrointestinal (GI) tract, where substances could more easily get expelled or excreted. For example, if a person were to swallow a chunk of dental amalgam, he or she would absorb only 10 percent of the mercury as it made its way through the stomach lining. The majority would be excreted by the bowels. However, if we took the same amount of amalgam and pulverized it, as is the case when we inhale it as a filling is being drilled out, we'd absorb 80 percent of that mercury via the lungs into our body.[48] So, breathing it in is eight times worse than swallowing it.

Once this material gets through the mucosal membranes or is inhaled into the lungs, it is more readily absorbed into other organs such as the brain, liver, kidneys, or into fatty tissue, where there is a diminished opportunity for the body to rid itself of the toxicity by, for instance, vomiting it up.

Dr. Dana Colson, a Toronto biological dentist, underscores the importance of maintaining an optimal state of health in the mouth as this contributes to better overall health. For example, people with diabetes with good oral health have better glucose readings, she notes. The mouth is the portal through which infections enter the rest of the body, making oral health and general health inseparable. We have more bacteria in our mouth compared to any animal mouth, and if oral bacteria gets into the rest of our body it can diminish our immune system and damage organs such as the heart and lungs. Oral bacteria has been found in pancreatic cancer, as well as in the brains of patients with Alzheimers and dementia. Dr. Colson says that bleeding gums are a doorway for bacteria and fungi to enter the rest of the body. Oral DNA testing can be helpful in determining if this is a problem that should be attended to.

The Connection between Oral Health and Intestinal Health
GAPS — that is, Gut and Psychology Syndrome — is described by Dr. Natasha Campbell-McBride.[49] She is a neurologist with training in

48   Lorscheider, F. L., Vimy, M. J., & Summers, A. O. (1995). Mercury exposure from "silver" tooth fillings: Emerging evidence questions a traditional dental paradigm. *Journal of the Federation of American Societies for Experimental Biology, 9*(44), 504-508. https://doi.org/10.1096/fasebj.9.7.7737458

49   Frisch, T. (2016, March 31). Interview: Dr. Natasha Campbell-McBride discusses the science behind GAPS, modern nutrition woes.

human nutrition who created a diet for healing a leaky gut. Leaky gut is characterized by holes in the gut, as some of the toxins pierce holes in the intestines. Campbell-McBride makes a convincing case that a large percentage of cancers and other chronic diseases come from poor gut health. She believes that two out of three cancers are caused by leaky gut, a condition that is missed by most practitioners. The good flora in our gut secrete good protein and good bacteria, but the bad flora secrete harmful toxins. Most of us are chronically exposed to low-dose toxins in the environment that, along with other stressors, such as emotional ones, can create free radicals in our bodies. Additionally, early over-consumption of dairy products and antibiotics, and poor nutrition generate toxins in the gut. These toxins escape the gut and get into the bloodstream, roaming the body, where, according to Dr. Campbell-McBride, they create harmful free radical damage. Once these poisons are in the bloodstream, it is more difficult to rid the body of them, whereas if they remained in the GI tract, we could reject or expel at least some of them. Additionally, with leaky gut it is more difficult to absorb bone-building materials like calcium, magnesium, and vitamin K2. This puts us at risk of poor bone health (osteoporosis), including the jawbone, the foundation of teeth. Raw food, which is often full of healthy nutrients, that may be dissolved or destroyed in the heating process during cooking, is encouraged for a cancer-free diet. However, it can be crunchy, and you need your teeth so you can chew and masticate the food adequately so it can be absorbed.

Amalgam Fillings and Mercury

Dental amalgam is comprised of 50% mercury, along with silver, copper, tin and zinc. According to some studies, mercury from dental amalgam fillings is the number one source of mercury exposure in humans, exceeding any residues we ingest from fish.[50] Mercury vapours, which are emitted by amalgam in fillings, do not remain

---

EcoFarmingDaily. Retrieved from http://ecofarmingdaily.com/ interview-natasha-campbell-mcbride-on-gut-health/

50   Mutter, J. (2011) Is dental amalgam safe for humans? The opinion of the scientific committee of the European Commission.

locked in the tooth. They are triggered when we drink hot liquids or eat, and are inhaled into the lungs.[51] If the temperature in the mouth is over 14 C, as is always the case, dental amalgam continues to vaporize and small amounts of the mercury leak out every day. Dr. Colson notes that mercury vapour is released by chewing things such as grains, nuts, seeds, and gum. Grinding and clenching teeth also releases mercury vapour. Jackson Emerson Abraham, of the US Army Environmental Hygiene Agency, along with his colleagues, conducted a study of 61 persons, some of whom had dental amalgam fillings, while others did not. They found that after chewing, people with amalgam fillings had almost twenty times more mercury vapour in their mouths than those without mercury fillings.[52]

Studies have linked dental amalgam to psychological and neurological problems, and to cardiac and immune system issues.[53] An increase in antibiotic resistant bacteria in oral and intestinal flora in primates has also been reported.[54] While silver amalgam fillings were once con-

Journal of Occupational Medicine Toxicology, 6(2). https://doi.org/10.1186/1745-6673-6-2

51 Cox, R. D., & Reinhardt, J. W. (1979). Chewing releases mercury from fillings. *Lancet, 313*(8123), 985-986. https://doi.org/10.1016/50140-6736(79)91773-2

52 Abraham, J. E., Svare, C. W., & Frank, C. W. (1984). The effect of dental amalgam restorations on blood mercury levels. *Journal of Dental Research, 63*(1), 71-73. https://doi.org/10.1177/00220345 840630011801

53 Just, A., & Kall, J. (2017, July 31). Seven common misconceptions about dental mercury. *International Academy of Oral Medicine & Toxicology*. Retrieved from https://files.iaomt.org/wp-content/uploads/Misconceptions-Mercury.pdf

54 Edlund, C., Björkman, L., Ekstrand, J., Sandborgh-Englund, G., & Nord, C. E. (1996). . Resistance of normal human micro-flora to mercury and antimicrobials after exposure to mercury from dental amalgam fillings, *Clinical Infectious Disease, 22*(6), 944-950. Retrieved from https://www.ncbi.nlm.nih.gov/pubmed/8783691

sidered adequate in the mouth, we are now exposed to many more chemicals in our environment such as pesticides, processed ingredients in food, and various other contaminants. We don't have the adaptability that we had several decades ago, and mercury in amalgam contributes to the chemical overload in the body, says Dr. Colson.

Removing Amalgam Fillings

If you are considering removal of amalgam, you could consult an IOAMT (International Academy of Oral Medicine and Toxicology) trained dentist. This organization is comprised of medical, dental and research professionals. It investigates and communicates safe science-based treatments to promote whole body health. In relation to amalgam fillings, it trains and certifies dentists to remove mercury safely and to employ healthy material as filler in root canals.

When deciding to remove amalgam fillings, it's important to ensure that mercury vapour is not inhaled, and that there is minimal absorption under the tongue or around its edges, and via the mucosal tissues. The amalgam removal procedure is very important because in 30 seconds the mercury vapours can affect your thyroid if you are not protected.

Since a rubber dam alone is insufficient when drilling mercury out, the dentist engages in a fairly elaborate procedure to ensure the removal is done safely for the patient. Some of the important steps are listed below:

- draping the patient with a plastic apron under the dental bib to cover their clothing,
- a dental dam to fit the tooth and prevent particles from entering the oral mucosa,
- charcoal, chlorella, a cotton roll and gauze are placed under the dam to deal with any leakage of particles or metals,
- patients face is draped under the dam with a liner,
- goggles for the eyes and a hair cap,
- oxygen through nasal masks,
- an air filtration system in the form of a mercury vapour ionizer in the room.

Dentists in Ontario are required by law to have a special system that recycles and safely disposes of amalgam waste.

Even if you use a safe protocol when removing amalgam fillings, there is still mercury in the body, either from the procedure or from previous build-up. If a person has leaky gut syndrome, this should be healed prior to the amalgam removal procedure. Collaboration with a health care team can ensure good results by attending to detoxification through diet and other means, such as supplementation. Holistic practitioners may recommend supplements, such as Vitamin C, that can aid in ridding the body of mercury after amalgam removal. Laboratory tests administered before and after amalgam removal can also help monitor your progress.[55]

Metallothionein is a protective metal-binding protein that is produced in the body when levels of zinc, selenium, histidine, and cysteine are sufficient. It can also aid in the process of ridding the body of any mercury. Studies on mice that were deficient in this protein may be relevant to the human experience. Researcher Minoru Yoshida, University of Tokyo School of International Health, and colleagues, delivered mercury concentrations to mice in dosages that are relevant to humans. They found that the mice who were deficient in this protein exhibited more anxiety and had poorer memory. They concluded that these results would likely also apply to humans.[56]

Glutathione, a master detoxifying molecule produced by the body that has anti-cancer and antioxidant properties, is one of our body's natural defences. It helps combat some of the detrimental effects of metal absorption. However, if the body's production is inadequate, supplements to help the body fend off any excess chemical assault may be necessary.

55 Coulson, D. G. (2012). A safe protocol for amalgam removal. *Journal of Environmental and Public Health, 7.* https://doi.org/10.1155/2012/517391

56 Yoshida, M., Watanabe, C., Horie, K., & Satoh, M. (2004). Susceptibility of metallothionein-null mice to the behavioural alterations caused by exposure to mercury vapour at human -relevant concentration. *Toxicological Sciences 80*(1), 69-73. https://doi.org/10.1016/j.toxlet.2004.11.001

Metal, Gold Inlays, Crowns and Braces

Dr. Colson notes that metal-free dentistry is a healthy option and can replace crowns made with metals. Gold crowns, porcelain fused to gold, semi-precious and non- precious metals like palladium or nickel all have large electromagnetic fields. When two different metals such as amalgam and gold touch each other in the mouth, they generate an electromagnetic field (EMF). While gold crowns may work in the mouth as long as there are no other metals, some gold does contain metal such as palladium. Metals in the mouth may interfere with the flow of overall body energy. Depending on an individual's particular sensitivity, this could cause extra stress on the cardiovascular, neurological or immune systems, says Dr. Coulson. She notes that black circular lines along the gum line of a tooth that has a crown suggest an electromagnetic field from the metals on that tooth.

Nickel is a harmful chemical that is used in the mouths of both children and adults in partial dentures and in stainless steel crowns. Nickel in the mouth is absorbed first into the mucosa, then enters the bloodstream. An article in the International Journal of Dentistry by Dr. David Keinan and fellow researchers calls for further investigation of the release of toxic metals such as nickel, chromium and iron used in dental work with children.[57] Palladium, another heavy metal and toxin used in metal crowns, has a high EMF. Heavy metals in the body can also displace essential minerals, such as calcium, magnesium and selenium and can lead to poor calcium absorption, thyroid dysfunction, and affect the immune system.[58] Discuss with your dentist whether this is a component of your crown.

---

57   Keinan, D., Mass, E., & Zilberman, U. (2010). Absorption of nickel, chromium and iron by the root surface of primary molars covered with stainless steel crowns. *International Journal of Dentistry, 2010.* https://doi.org/10.1155/2010/326124

58   Rau, T., & Vizkelety, J. An interdisciplinary approach of doctors & dentists at the Paracelsus Clinic. *Marion*

Clear aligners which are made of plastic and are Bisphenol A- free are a healthier choice than metal braces for people with metal sensitivities, says Dr. Colson.

What to Do When Told You Need a Root Canal

A dentist's job is to provide you with enough information to make an informed decision on how to proceed. If a dentist recommends having a root canal, many holistic dentists suggest that a person get a second opinion. Sometimes the tooth is not dead or infected. If there is only an inflammation, a dentist may be able to save it by injecting homeopathic anti-inflammatory substances into the tooth tissue. If the root canal tooth can't be saved, there are two possible routes: one is to have the root canal done and keep the tooth. The other route is to have the tooth in question extracted.

If a root canal is performed, the infection in the tooth is cleaned, disinfected and then sealed. However, many articles report that root canals remain chronically infected as it is impossible to adequately clean out the millions of side canals, or dentin tubules. Studies show that various types of yeast, such as Candida albicans and anaerobic gram-negative bacteria, populate the root canal and dentin tubules of the tooth.[59] Some mainstream medical journals say that it is impossible to remove all the infection or protect the tooth from subsequent reinfection. New technology and research show that Waterlase and ozone can help sterilize the canals. Antibiotics are helpful in eliminating infections in the bone and around the tooth. However, they may not reach the tubules as there is no more blood supply to the tooth, meaning that the blood that would otherwise carry the antibiotics cannot get inside the canals. Any residual toxins are able to travel

Institute. Retrieved from https://www.marioninstitute.org/metals-and-heavy-metals-a-risk-for-our-health/

59 Waltimo, T. M. T., Sen, B. H., Meurman, J. H., Ørstavik, D., & Haapasalo, M. P. P. (2003). Yeasts in apical periodontitis. *Critical Reviews in Oral Biology and Medicine, 14*(2), 128. https://doi.org/10.1177/154411130301400206

down through the gum ligament, bone and bloodstream, and on to organs and tissue around the body. These harmful bacteria circulating in the blood stream colonize themselves in organs and tissue elsewhere in the body. The immune system is then permanently "on call," chronically fighting a low-grade infection, and ready to trigger an inflammatory response somewhere in the body. This may manifest itself in a multitude of ways — for instance joints, valves, some say breast tissue, and so on.

> Waterlase dentistry is a new technology that employs laser energy and water to perform dental procedures faster and more comfortably, mostly without the need for anaesthesia.

Dr. Colson asserts that if the nerve of the tooth has not been infected but there is extensive decay, the application of either silver diamine fluoride or ozone, or both, may eliminate the need for a root canal. Re-mineralizing the softened decay close to the pulp in this way helps prevent many root canal treatments and also helps the nerve and blood supply to the tooth remain vital.

Removing a Root Canal; Managing the Gap with Implants, Partial Dentures and Bridges

Some holistic dentists recommend removing the tooth since a treated root canal may continue to produce toxins such as yeast and endotoxins, which may cause chronic low-grade infections. The infection and toxins can circulate around the body and affect not only the tooth but distant organs, as described above.[60] If you do remove a root canal there are several options for dealing with the area that remains after the tooth extraction.

Upon removal of the tooth, the dentist should scrape out the infection in the jawbone, ensuring as much as possible, that no remnants,

---

60   Kulacz, R., & Levy, T. E. (2014). *The toxic tooth: How a root canal could be making you sick.* Henderson, NV: Medfox Publishing.

called granulation tissue, remains. If there are pockets of infection left behind, antibiotics or the body may not rectify this.

Once the tooth is out, you can choose to either go without a tooth, have a partial denture, an implant, or a fixed bridge. Partial dentures usually contain chromium and cobalt. Gold, titanium or a metal-free partial denture are better options. With partial dentures, a monomer-free denture made from acrylic or thermoplastic, and in some cases even employing some silicone, may be best. Clear acrylic with no colour may be less toxic and more biocompatible for denture users, as colouring agents can be toxic. Some studies show monomers may be carcinogenic, and small amounts can leak out of acrylic. Adequate lab processing can rectify this.[61,62] Blood serum biocompatibility tests are available to verify which substance is best for you.

If you have teeth on either side of the area where the teeth are missing, another option is a fixed bridge. You do have to reduce the two teeth on either side, but less reduction is necessary today due to non-metal materials now available. Dr. Colson says that Maryland style bridges may be possible, depending on how your teeth connect. You should discuss this with your dentist.

A third option is a dental implant. When you lose a tooth and do not replace it with a dental implant, you can lose bone around the tooth in the first year due to the way it heals. A dental implant exercises the jawbone and stops it from disintegrating. Chewing with the implant exerts force on the jawbone, providing physical stimulation. Titanium implants have been most commonly used in the past, and they are biocompatible. In the last few years in Canada, biocompatible

---

61 Gosavi, S. S., Gosavi, S. Y., Alla, R. K. (2010). Local and systemic effects of unpolymerised monomers. *Dental Research Journal, 7*(2), 82-87. Retrieved from https://www.ncbi.nlm.nih.gov/pmc/articles/PMC3177373/

62 Leggat, P. A., & Kudjarune, U. (2003). Toxicity of methyl methacrylate in dentistry. *International Dental Journal, 53*(3), 126-131. https://doi.org/10.1111/j.1875-595X.2003.tb00736.x

ceramic implants made of zirconia have become available in some dental offices. After a few months of healing on the cellular level, the bone solidifies around the implant, and the dentist can then place a crown on top. One of the big advantages with implants is that the dentist can remove the tooth and place the implant in place the same day if there is no infection in the bone.

Some medical practitioners believe that an implant is a foreign body, and some foreign bodies generate inflammation. Most dentists believe that this is not a problem with implants. However, some dentists do suggest caution for people who are smokers, uncontrolled diabetics, or have compromised immune systems, such as people who have had cancer in the last 10 years. In such cases, the implant may not integrate into the jawbone.

Dr. Colson recommends doing a bio-compatibility test (mentioned above) before inserting a dental implant, especially in patients who have particular chemical sensitivities, an impaired immune system, or any serious illness. While zirconia has less of an electromagnetic field than titanium, it still generates metal energy, she says, a factor that needs to be considered in the overall mouth health of the patient. Additionally, about 80% of implants still require some modification or correction over a lifetime.

Night guards

Dr. Colson says night guards, also known as biteplates, are very important as they can protect one's teeth from excess wear and fracture. They enable our temporomandibular joint (TMJ) to be comfortable, which is turn allows for relaxed facial muscles. This contributes to a stress free mouth, which can help minimize stress overall in the body. Some new materials used in night guards can leak monomers. Monomers can be toxic if not processed properly as they can release Bisphenol A (BPA). A night guard, which is constructed so that its softens in hot water prior to placing in one's mouth and then hardens in the mouth, may leak monomers. Some people are sensitive and may have allergies to monomers. It's important to discuss which night guard material might be best for you with your dentist. A blood serum biocompatibility test can also be helpful in determining this.

Bisphenol A (BPA) is a chemical that is added to many commercial products. It can bind to hormone receptors in the body, including estrogen receptors and adversely affect their function.

The Connection between Mouth Health and Breast Cancer

With respect to cancer and dentistry, breast cancer is especially interesting because breasts have a lot of adipose tissue and heavy metals, like mercury, have an affinity for fatty tissue. Studies have found a smorgasbord of heavy metals used in dentistry, such as nickel, chromium, cadmium, and mercury, in the breast tissue of women with breast cancer.[63] Additionally, some articles in mainstream dental journals report that formally inspected root canals may be chronically infected.[64] Traditional Chinese medicine describes this process in relation to meridians. It notes that the teeth are on acupuncture meridians related to different organs in the body.

In Chinese medicine, meridians are the overall energy distribution system in the body. Organs and tissue in one part of the body are connected by meridians to other parts of the body.

The connection between teeth and acupuncture meridians was reported by Dr. Reinhold Voll, anatomy professor and acupuncturist in

---

63   Ionescu, J. G., Novotny, J., Stejskal, V., Lätsch, A., Blaurock-Busch, E., & Eisenmann-Klein, M. (2007). Increased levels of transition metals in breast cancer tissue. *Neuro Endocrinology Letters, 27*(Suppl. 1), 36-39. Retrieved from https://www.researchgate.net/publication/6979212_Increased_levels_of_transition_metals_in_breast_cancer_tissue

64   Haapasalo, M., Udnæs, T., & Endal, U. (2004) Persistent, recurrent and acquired infection of the root canal system post-treatment. *Endodontic Topics, 6*(2). https://doi.org/10.1111/j.1601-1546.2003.00041.x

the fifties.[65] Dr. Voll noted that unhealthy teeth could interfere with the energy flow along the relevant meridians, thereby affecting the health of organs or tissues on the corresponding meridian. Similarly, the process could take place in the reverse since every major organ is linked via meridians to a specific tooth. For example, some back teeth on the upper jaw are on the breast meridian, and anecdotally, people will often have cancer on the same side as a root canal, possibly related to chronic tooth infection. Dr. Voll researched and perfected an innovative testing method known as the electroacupuncture according to Voll (EAV), or electro-dermal screening test. This test uses electrical current to measure the flow of energy through meridians in the body, that is channels through which the body's energy passes, connecting organs and tissue. The EAV indicates the health of the meridian and the associated organs and tissue. If there was inflammation along the meridian, the EAV would be able to detect this by indicating a higher than average flow of energy along that meridian. A dentist who I spoke to reported anecdotally that many patients who came to his office with breast cancer also had issues such as infected teeth, root canals, hidden bone infections, toxic restorations and metal implants on the same side as the breast cancer.

Fluoride and Health

There are many references to fluoride as a carcinogen.[66] Some studies have linked osteosarcoma in males under 20 to fluoride in water. Some studies report that fluoride, when ingested, accumulates in the bone, possibly causing mutations at certain vulnerable time periods in a young male's life.[67] Some dentists believe children should not swallow the fluoride rinses employed after dental work or eat for half

---

65   Kidd, R. F. (2005). *Neural therapy: Applied neurophysiology and other topics.* Custom printers of Renfrew Ltd.

66   Woffinden, B. (2005, June 12). Fluoride water "causes cancer". *The Observer.* Retrieved from https://www.theguardian.com/society/2005/jun/12/medicineandhealth.genderissues

67   Bassin, E. B., Wypij, D., Davis, R. B., & Mittleman, M. A. (2006). Age-specific fluoride exposure in drinking water and osteosarcoma

an hour after a dental treatment that is followed by a fluoride rinse. It is used in small amounts in water to prevent tooth decay. It can make bones more brittle, and in areas with high fluoride water content, it can affect the development of the enamel.[68] Many believe that a diet free of natural and processed sugars and good oral hygiene can prevent decay.

Cavities can be controlled by managing the level of acidity in the body through diet. Certain foods, such as sugars and some grains, increase the bacterial content in the mouth. This, in turn, increases the acidity in the mouth, which leads to an increase in tooth decay. It is possible to purchase litmus paper and monitor oral acidity levels. The acid level is determined by taking readings of saliva three times a day (morning, midday, and evening) at least twenty minutes after eating or tooth brushing for fourteen consecutive days. Acidity in the body fluctuates during the day. If the saliva is too acidic, you may be more at risk for cavities. To aid in rectifying this, you need to alkalinize your diet more, thereby increasing the pH (the acid/alkaline balance) in the body. The optimal level is a reading of 7.0.

Lemon water is acidic outside the body, but alkalizes when digested by the body and is therefore good for overall health. Alkalizing the body contributes to oxygenating cells and fighting inflammation, says Dr. Colson. Cancer cells are less able to survive in an anaerobic, that is oxygen-free, environment. Excessive consumption of lemon water can cause erosion of the tooth enamel, so she advises brushing teeth before drinking lemon water. Rinsing your mouth with large amounts of water immediately after drinking the lemon water will neutralize the acid and will also help prevent the erosion.

(United States). *Cancer Causes Control, 17*(4), 421-428. Retrieved from https://www.ncbi.nlm.nih.gov/pubmed/16596294

68   Everett, E. T. (2011). Fluoride's effects on the formation of teeth and bones and the influence of genetics. *Journal of Dental Research, 90*(5), 552-560. https://doi.org/10.1177/0022034510384626

CHAPTER 12

A Summary of the Practitioners Perspectives

In this chapter, I provide a short summary of each practitioner's perspective on cancer prevention, treatment, and ongoing management. This will give you an overview of what they believe is important and available. The summary of biological dentistry offers a more general synopsis of how mouth health relates to overall health, which includes the immune system and the functioning of various organs. Though some of the advice that one professional offers may be at odds with another professional, it is important for you, the reader, to be as informed as possible about all perspectives. Then you are able to choose what makes sense to you.

Sat Dharam Kaur, naturopath, encourages cancer prevention and management with supplements, regular blood monitoring, and urine and saliva tests to monitor insulin-like growth factors and insulin levels. She also employs strategies to rid the body of the bad estrogen and to deal with liver toxicity.

- Eating a plant-based diet and cutting out sugar is a crucial place to start when managing breast cancer. Supplementation with, for example, vitamin D3, vitamin C, NAC, probiotics, curcumin, and flax seeds helps support the liver in flushing out toxins and lowering estrogen levels.

- The damage radiation does may be worse than chemo, but if you opt for radiation, you can get some protection with certain herbs, supplements, and antioxidants such as miso, kelp, and vitamin C, which reduce radioactive molecules. Antioxidants such as vitamin C, glutathione, and alpha lipoic acid (a synthetic version of lipoic acid that is an antioxidant vital to cellular energy reproduction) are free radical scavengers and can be taken during or after radiation.
- Herbs, mushrooms, and antioxidants can also reduce the free radical load and keep the immune system as strong as possible during chemo, and antioxidants can minimize the side effects.
- To prevent recurrence or metastasis, monitor iron levels, tumour markers such as CEA and CA 15-3, blood stickiness with fibrinogen and fibrin d-dimers, and signs of inflammation in the body with C-reactive protein levels.
- Minimize stress through practices like meditation, yoga, and exercise.

Dr. Alvin Pettle, gynecologist, says that when the ovaries shut down during menopause, the adrenal glands need to take over. However, when stress has depleted the adrenals and DHEA is low, they are unable to take over this function. This causes hypoxic cells, that is oxygen starved cells, which can cause abnormal cells to multiply, elevating breast cancer risk. Progesterone, Pettle says, is the body's natural balancing hormone, and counters the effect of ovarian imbalance by keeping estrogen in check. Some believe that breast cancer surgery is more successful when progesterone is high and estrogen low. Lori, who was interviewed for this book and had consulted Dr. Pettle, recalls that when she was diagnosed with breast cancer, she discovered this research and then sought a surgeon who considered this in scheduling her surgery.

- A woman's path to breast cancer is multifactorial and is determined by genetics, environmental factors, diet, nutrition, and hormonal imbalances.

- Keeping the level of the stress hormone cortisol low is paramount. To prevent and treat breast cancer, one also needs to consider the hormonal imbalance in the ovaries, thyroid and adrenal glands. Administering DHEA drops under the tongue and estriol cream applied inside the vagina, as well as progesterone cream (which helps protect against estrogen dominance), is a big step towards harmonizing hormones. In Dr. Pettle's opinion, hormonal interventions such as DHEA, progesterone, and estriol are acceptable for women with breast cancer, as long as they are closely monitored.
- Chemotherapy and radiation may be more destructive than curative.
- Tamoxifen carries a risk of side effects that may cancel any benefits obtained in suppressing estrogen production in this way. Instead, estrogen production can be suppressed by rectifying hormonal imbalances with, for instance, DHEA drops, estriol cream, making dietary changes, exercising, increasing water intake, and taking supplements, such as Myomins.
- Thermograms are a good early diagnostic option and could be used in conjunction with other screening devices, such as ultrasound. Mammograms may not be a good screening device, as they carry many risks. They irradiate, crush, and can traumatize to the breast.

Dr. Alex Mostovoy, homeopath, employs thermograms, a safe diagnostic tool that evaluates the level of inflammation in the breast, a possible precursor for a tumour. Thermograms do not have any harmful side effects, unlike mammography. According to Dr. Stephen Malthouse, a medical doctor and past president of the Canadian Complementary Medical Association, homeopathy may be an inexpensive, convenient, and safe intervention that contributes to well-being and integrates well with conventional medicine.

- Preventive work, including dealing with unexpressed trauma, environmental pollutants, diet, and exercise, is crucial in order to prevent cancer, as well as its recurrences, and to prevent many chronic conditions that often precede cancer.

- Thermograms are a safe screening tool and early warning system for women in high-risk groups. They are benign and non-invasive, and can pick up inflammatory disease in breast tissue, which may be a precursor of cancer. They can minimize radiation and biopsies.
- Surgery, without dealing with the causes of the cancer on a systemic level, may only predispose the patient to developing cancer elsewhere.
- Addressing an individual on a psycho-emotional, biophysical, and biochemical level will help his or her body to self-correct.

Dr. Fred Hui, integrative physician, highlights the remarkable results achieved by some medical practitioners around the globe, some of whom have been silenced despite the documented beneficial effects of their treatments. Some practitioners continue on a quiet path to effecting recovery in those patients who happen to stumble upon them.

- Hormonal imbalance — as indicated by such symptoms as heavy periods, premenstrual syndrome, and tender breasts — must be properly addressed. Progesterone administered topically can moderate the estrogen overload that creates an imbalance and serve as a preventative measure for breast cancer. Supplementation with topical bio-identical hormones such as BiEst or transdermal estriol cream can help create a healthy balance of estrogen and serve as a preventative measure for breast cancer.
- Twenty milligrams of melatonin at bedtime in breast cancer patients can reset the body clock, improve sleep, and contribute to a strong immune system. Arimidex and tamoxifen can be useful in suppressing excess estrogen production. Intravenous vitamin C can contribute to apoptosis (death) of cancer cells.
- After chemo and radiation, the body can recover and be nourished back to health through attention to the state of the adrenal glands, thyroid, and kidneys.

Dr. Ahmad Nasri, homeopath and naturopath, offers various treatments, including intravenous administration of vitamins, minerals, and biological modulators that can be effective in causing cancer cell death, particularly with stage I and II breast cancer. Dr. Nasri's protocol combines oral supplementation and dietary interventions at home with intravenous treatments in the clinic.

- Surgery to remove a malignant tumour generally improves treatment outcome, but for patients who refuse surgery, lesions can remain stable as long as their immune systems remains strong, keeping the tumours in check.
- Alternative treatments can work well with stage I and II cancers, in lieu of chemo and radiation, and should at least be employed initially because they avoid the collateral damage of chemotherapy and radiation. With stage III and IV cancers, alternative treatments can be used in combination with conventional treatments, and can ameliorate some of the detrimental side effects of these harsh treatments.
- While many allopathic doctors argue that powerful antioxidants taken during chemo interfere with its effectiveness, many studies have shown to the contrary. These studies show that there is a synergy between some chemo agents and alternative treatments, and that alternative treatments can actually augment the beneficial effects of chemo.
- If a patient is anaemic, this must be dealt with before chemotherapy, because chemo will further worsen anemia.
- IgG and IgA tests are antibody tests that help determine a person's sensitivity, or intolerance to certain foods. These tests are helpful in planning an individualized diet and provide information on which foods will enhance a person's immune-system functioning.

Dr. Charles Hayter, radiation oncologist, has commemorated courageous oncologist Vera Peters in a play. She fought the surgical lobby in Toronto in the seventies, challenging the belief that radical mastectomy was superior to lumpectomy in the treatment of early stage breast cancer. Many years later, her research contributed to policy changes away from performing blanket mastectomies to lumpectomy, as appropriate.

- Giving patients a voice and choice in their treatment and respecting their wishes is paramount.
- Many conventional treatments have their origin in non-conventional ones; therefore, the division between the two may be artificial. Scientific evidence is needed to support all interventions, including integrative and alternative treatments for cancer.

Dr. Shailendra Verma, medical oncologist, urges further evidence-based research by alternative and integrative practitioners to promote more collaboration across professions, in particular with naturopaths.

- Surgery for breast cancer to remove the primary cancer is crucial. Following that, a woman should have a careful and informed discussion regarding the benefits and risks of adjuvant therapy.
- The time is right for both conventional and complementary health care professionals to collaborate on research and on clinical interventions with patients. Collectively, all professionals can help to move patients into a more self-sufficient role, where they are less dependent on drugs and engage in behaviours such as stress reduction, weight management, and careful monitoring of diet. All of these methods can help the body to heal and reduce the risk of recurrence.

Several **biological dentists** who were interviewed report that oral health and overall health are inseparable.

- Metal-free dentistry is good for overall health.
- Dental materials used in the mouth can enter the rest of the body through mucosal membranes, blood, or if inhaled into the lungs.
- Mercury in amalgam fillings continues to off gas in the mouth and has been linked to health issues in many studies. When

removing amalgam fillings, a strict protocol should be adhered to so that no mercury enters the body.

- Root canals are often difficult to adequately clean, and some say remain chronically infected which can affect distant organs.
- Implants can work well for some people as they exercise the bone and prevent further disintegration. However, some dentists recommend caution when considering them for people with, for example, compromised immune systems such as some cancer patients.

Part III

A Path to Recovery

CHAPTER 13

The Well-Worn Path

In this chapter, I highlight scientific research data related to breast cancer prevention and treatments that patients may not be presented with when facing choices about a treatment path, or when choosing preventive measures.

Current Breast Cancer Diagnosis and Treatment: The Uncertainties

While women are encouraged to regularly palpate their breasts to detect malignant tumours as early as possible, there remains uncertainty about the implications of any that are found. For instance, it is often unclear whether a particular breast cancer tumour will respond to treatment, and therefore difficult to decide which treatment would be best. The question of whether the tumour would be life-threatening if it were left untreated is also significant.[69]

Following a breast cancer diagnosis, a patient will be offered some combination of surgery, chemotherapy, radiation or hormonal therapy. Several factors will influence which of these treatments will be viewed as necessary. These factors include the nuclear grade of the tumour,

---

69   Brenner, B. (2009). New Study Points to Problems with
      Breast Cancer Screening. *The Source, winter 2009*(108).
      Retrieved from https://bcaction.org/2009/12/21/
      new-study-points-to-problems-with-breast-cancer-screening/

the differentiation grade, the size of the tumour and extent of spread, and the hormonal status. They are explained more fully below :

- The nuclear grade of the tumour describes how similar the nuclei of the cancer cell is to the nuclei of the normal breast cell. This determination is given a grading from 1 to 3. A nuclear grade of 1 suggests the nuclei are the most similar to nuclei of normal cancer cells. A higher nuclear grade usually suggests a more abnormal nuclei and more aggressive tumour cells.

- The differentiation grade ranges from "poorly differentiated" through "moderately differentiated" to "well differentiated". Well differentiated suggests the cells look almost like normal cells, and tend to grow slowly and are less likely to spread. Poorly differentiated cells tend to grow more quickly and are more likely to spread.

- The size of the tumour and extent of spread is labelled in Stages 1 to 4. Under 2 centimetres in size with no nodal involvement is considered stage 1. Stage 2 refers to 2 to 5 centimetres in size with limited or no nodal involvement, and is considered to be early breast cancer. Both stages 1 and 2 are believed to have the best prognosis. Stage III is determined by a combination of the size of the tumour and the extent of the spread, specifically if the malignant cells have spread to the nodes. Stage IV indicates the cancer has spread to other parts of the body.

- Hormonal status indicates whether the tumour is estrogen positive or negative, or progesterone positive or negative. Estrogen feeds cancer and progesterone balances estrogen, so hormonal status will determine whether hormonal therapy, such as tamoxifen or aromatase inhibitors that suppress estrogen production, will be offered post-surgery.

- HER 2 (human epidermal growth factor receptor 2) is a gene. When it malfunctions it can cause breast cells to grow and divide uncontrollably. HER 2 positive breast cancers may have a poorer outcome than those that are HER 2 negative because they tend to grow faster, are more likely to spread, and tend to return.

The current "one size fits all" approach to treatment, where treatment is determined by some combination of the above factors, has increasingly come under criticism as it does not tailor treatment to the biology of each tumour.

This may be a more important factor in determining whether a tumour will metastasize. One of the determinants of breast cancer prognosis has traditionally been the size of the tumour; however, this does not necessarily accurately predict outcome. A small tumour may have a great potential to metastasize, while a large tumour may not.[70] Therefore, when a woman receives a diagnosis of, for example, stage IV cancer, meaning her tumour is significantly larger than a stage 1 tumour, she may feel more frightened and less hopeful based on the tumour characteristics. In actuality, the larger tumour may not metastasize, while a smaller one might.

In a 2016 article on the anatomy of cancer in the New York Times, Siddhartha Mukherjee highlights the difficulties in the successful treatment of cancer. He notes that no other human disease is known to be as "genetically heterogeneous" as cancer is.[71] These unlimited variations of the cancer cell, may, he says, explain the different responses to treatment. He points out that the standard protocols have in the past categorized cancer based on where it is located in the body. And likewise, the chemotherapy used to treat it has also been determined by where the cancer is located in the body, and has rarely been altered for individual patients and their particular cancer. He mentions two drugs that have been in use in the last couple of decades that target a very specific genetic mutation in lung cancer and leukemia. If patients with these two cancers have a different mutation, and many do, these drugs are of no benefit.

---

70   Esserman, L. J., Thompson, I. M., Reid, B., Nelson, P., Ransohoff, D. F., Welch, H. G., ... Srivastava, S. (2014). Addressing overdiagnosis and overtreatment in cancer: A prescription for change. *Lancet Oncology, 15*(6), 234-242. https://doi.org/10.1016/S1470-2045(13)70598-9

71   Mukherjee, S. (2016, May 15). Doctors without borders: The new anatomy of cancer. *The New York Times Magazine*, p. 46.

Given the real uncertainty related to tumour characteristics and outcome, and the treatments that are prescribed based on these uncertain characteristics, I believe it is important to more critically examine some of the most common screening tools, such as mammography, MRI, and ultrasound, as well as treatments that are often prescribed following a breast cancer diagnosis, such as mastectomy, chemotherapy, and radiation. I will also discuss thermograms, a safe alternative to screening mammography. Critical evaluation of these tools and interventions by doctors and other health care professionals is too often lacking. When one is suddenly faced with a diagnosis and feels pressured to make quick choices about treatment, those women who choose to follow a course that makes sense to them outside of the customary allopathic route may be left feeling nervous and uncertain. If they are accused by conventional oncologists of not doing what the doctor believes they should do to regain their health, they may also feel delinquent. I personally had this experience when I was reprimanded by an administrative staff member of the oncologist who was treating me early on in the course of my breast cancer. When I said that I did not wish to continue with tamoxifen, she reprimanded me for not "following their protocol". This reaction hastened my departure from her care as I did not feel welcome if I made choices about my treatment that she did not agree with. I have also heard about people who are sometimes even refused care by oncologists for not following the standard protocol. This attitude on the part of certain doctors is unwarranted and harmful given the mixed scientific data and the uncertainty that exists in relation to breast cancer treatment and cure.

Screening Mammography

Mammography serves as a major screening tool for breast cancer, yet its utility as such is controversial. Unlike diagnostic mammography, which may be used along with other tools to help confirm suspicious lumps, screening mammography is performed at regular intervals in asymptomatic women. This protocol was initiated to impact mortality by finding and treating more early stage cancers, thereby reducing the incidence of advanced cancers. Though massive mammography screening has resulted in an increase in the detection of early stage cancers, it has not resulted in fewer advanced cancers, nor has it had an impact on mortality.[72] In addition, the resulting overdiagnosis has led to overtreatment in women, which can bring a host of unnecessary difficulties to the patient. A mammogram squeezes, irradiates and traumatizes the breast while performing its function, which is an added hazard. Some of the pitfalls of screening mammography are explored further below.

A 2014 Canadian study that examined the impact of screening mammography on mortality over a 20 year period in more than 50,000 women aged 40 to 49 found that its impact was insignificant. The results indicated that whether or not you screen a woman in her forties with mammography, her chances of dying of breast cancer before the age of 60 were approximately equal.[73] Based on their results and his own, Gilbert Welch asserted that mammography screening had no impact on breast cancer mortality, and that one in five invasive breast cancers detected by mammography constituted overdiagnosis.[74,75,76]

72 Bleyer, A., & Welch, H. G. (2012). Effects of three decades of screening mammography on breast cancer incidence. *New England Journal of Medicine, 367*, 1998-2005. https://doi.org/10.1056/NEJMoa1206809

73 Narod, S., Sun, P., Wall, C., Baines, C., & Miller, A. B. (2014). Impact of screening mammography on mortality from breast cancer before age 60 in women 40-49 years of age. *Current Oncology, 21*(5), 217-221. https://doi.org/10.3747/co.21.2067

74 Bleyer, A., & Welch, H. G. (2012). Effects of three decades of screening mammography on breast cancer incidence. *New England Journal of Medicine, 367*, 1998-2005. https://doi.org/10.1056/NEJMoa1206809

75 Miller, A. B., Wall, C., Baines, C. J., Sun, P., To, T., Narod, S. A. (2014). Twenty five year follow-up for breast cancer incidence and mortality of the Canadian National Breast Screening Study: Randomised screening trial. *British Medical Journal, 2014*, 348-366. https://doi.org/10.1136/bmj.g366

76 PBS NewsHour. (2014, February 12). *Debating the value and effectiveness of mammograms* [Video

Gilbert Welch, MD, professor of medicine at Dartmouth Institute of Health Policy and Clinical Practice, is an author of numerous scientific papers and a book on mammography, overdiagnosis, and breast cancer.

Early stage cancers are increasingly found with mammography screening, and include both DCIS, a non-spreading cancer, and some invasive cancers. Yet, many early stage cancers may not need treatment, as they may never grow, or may even regress.[77] Welch says that some lesions may be a cellular abnormality that could not only potentially regress, but might even disappear. However, doctors feel they must treat cancer such as DCIS or atypical cells, once found, whether or not they are likely to spread.[78]

According to Dr. John Lee, the increase in DCIS diagnoses has made the overall breast cancer cure rate seem better than it really is, as for the most part this is a non-spreading cancer. DCIS is contained within the duct and "in situ" means that there is no penetration of the deeper layers of the skin.[79] Prior to mammography screening, DCIS lesions represented 3 percent of all cancers found. Now they account

---

file]. Retrieved from https://www.pbs.org/video/debating-the-value-and-effectiveness-of-mammograms-1399501305/

77 Zahl, P-H., Gøtzsche, P. C., Mæhlen, J. (2011). Natural history of breast cancers detected in the Swedish mammography screening programme: A cohort study. *Lancet Oncology, 12*(12), 1118-1124. https://doi.org/10.1016/S1470-2045(11)70250-9

78 Welch, H. G., & Frankel, B. A. (2011). Likelihood that a woman with screen-detected breast cancer has had her "life saved" by that screening. *Archives of Internal Medicine, 171*(22), 2043-2046. https://doi.org/10.1001/archinternmed.2011.476

79 Lee, J. R., Zava, D., & Hopkins, V. (2005). *What your doctor might not tell you about Breast cancer: How hormone balance can help save your life*. New York, NY: Warner Books, p. 52.

for 20 to 25 percent of "screen-detected breast cancers."[80] In a 2009 meta-analysis of seven breast cancer studies, the Nordic Cochrane Centre in Copenhagen, reported that breast cancer screening led to a 30 percent rate of overdiagnosis and overtreatment.[81]

The Nordic Cochrane Centre in Copenhagen is an arm of a well-respected international network of individuals and institutes that maintains and distributes systematic reviews of effects of health care.

In a landmark study in 2014, Laura Esserman, professor of surgery and radiology at the University of California, San Francisco, and a prolific researcher in this field, reported that the extent of overdiagnosis of what she calls "indolent lesions" (that is, those lesions that are currently labelled as cancer but are low risk and, if left untreated, likely will not cause any harm) is underappreciated, and ranges from 20 to 30 percent. This applies not only to DCIS, in which abnormal cells are found in the lining of the milk ducts, but also to some invasive cancers.[82] These results were in line with the earlier Danish report.

The majority of women diagnosed with DCIS are in their forties. Once they receive this diagnosis, they may then undergo any number of invasive treatments, such as surgery (which would include

---

80   Esserman, L. J., & Yau, C. (2015). Rethinking the standard for ductal carcinoma in situ treatment. *Journal of American Medical Association, 7*, 881-883. https://doi.org/10.1001/jamaoncol.2015.2607

81   Jorgensen, K., & Gøtzsche, P. C. (2009). Overdiagnosis in publicly organized mammography screening programmes: Systematic review of incidence trends. *British Medical Journal, 2009*, 339. https://doi.org/10.1136/bmj.b2587

82   Esserman, L. J., Thompson, I. M., Reid, B., Nelson, P., Ransohoff, D. F., Welch, H. G., ... Srivastava, S. (2014). Addressing overdiagnosis and overtreatment in cancer: A prescription for change. *Lancet Oncology, 15*(6), 234-242. https://doi.org/10.1016/S1470-2045(13)70598-9

lumpectomy or mastectomy), chemotherapy and radiation. In the U.S., approximately 50,000 healthy women per year are diagnosed with DCIS. The Danish researchers mentioned above reported that in a sample of two thousand women screened regularly, only one woman will benefit from early detection, while two hundred women will get false positive results. Once diagnosed, they may follow an anxiety-provoking and fear-laden path that may involve multiple unnecessary medical interventions, such as lumpectomy, mastectomy, chemotherapy and/or radiation. This might leave them with chronic pain, disfigurement, and a sense of themselves as chronically ill. This outcome would result in mammography harming ten times more women due to overdiagnosis and overtreatment than it helps.[83] Welch reported that over a period of ten years, half of all women screened will receive false alarms. Until a tumour is finally confirmed as benign, a patient may be called back for multiple tests which may leave a patient feeling physically and psychologically battered.[84]

Autopsy studies examining a sample of women age 40 to 54 who died from causes other than breast cancer found that 37 percent of those women had lesions of invasive and non-invasive cancers. These results suggested that the women examined in these studies died with cancer, but not from cancer, and their cancers had no implications for their overall health.[85] A recent Scandinavian study examined the course of invasive cancers in about 230,000 women in Norway and

83   Gøtzsche, P. C., & Nielsen, M. (2011). Screening for breast cancer with mammography. *Cochrane Database Systematic Reviews, 1.* https://doi.org/10.1002/14651858.CD001877.pub4

84   Welch, H. G. (2015, July 19). When screening is bad for a woman's health. *Los Angeles Times.* Retrieved from http://www.latimes.com/opinion/op-ed/la-oe-welch-harms-of-screening-mammograms-20150719-story.html

85   Jorgensen, K., & Gøtzsche, P. C. (2009). Overdiagnosis in publicly organized mammography screening programmes: Systematic review of incidence trends. *British Medical Journal, 2009,* 339. https://doi.org/10.1136/bmj.b2587

Sweden. It found that about 20 percent of certain invasive cancers, if left alone, spontaneously regressed.[86]

Overdiagnosis also generates a climate of fear related to the escalating numbers of cancers being found. This causes an increase in demand for screening, which subsequently results in more diagnosis of DCIS. And yet there is only a 5 percent chance of a DCIS lesion turning into an invasive cancer over a ten-year period.[87] Many believe that treating DCIS with radical measures is generally not necessary.[88] Esserman likens the overtreatment of DCIS to conducting heart surgery when a patient comes into the office with high cholesterol.[89]

Though cancer tumour size has been a standard marker of prognosis, it does not necessarily predict a particular outcome of cancer accurately. Malcolm Gladwell, in an article called "The Picture Problem," cites various researchers who claim that we overestimate the significance of tumour size, and that the biology of a particular cancer at the time it is removed may be more predictive of whether it will metastasize than its size. Mammography may miss small tumours that may carry a genetic program causing them to metastasize early, while picking up large tumours that could be found with less invasive methods and may not necessarily metastasize. Mammograms

86   Zahl, P-H., Gøtzsche, P. C., Mæhlen, J. (2011). Natural history of breast cancers detected in the Swedish mammography screening programme: A cohort study. *Lancet Oncology, 12*(12), 1118-1124. https://doi.org/10.1016/S1470-2045(11)70250-9

87   Orenstein, P. (2013, April 25). Our feel-good war on breast cancer. *New York Times*. Retrieved from https://www.nytimes.com/2013/04/28/magazine/our-feel-good-war-on-breast-cancer.html

88   O'Conner, S. (2015, October 1). Why doctors are rethinking breast cancer treatment. *Time Health 186*(14). Retrieved from http://time.com/4057310/breast-cancer-overtreatment/

89   Orenstein, P. (2013, April 25). Our feel-good war on breast cancer. *New York Times*. Retrieved from https://www.nytimes.com/2013/04/28/magazine/our-feel-good-war-on-breast-cancer.html

also tend to pick up cancers that grow slowly, because slow-growing cancers leave detectable calcium deposits (calcifications), but may miss cancers that do more harm. For instance, one interesting study examined tumours of 429 women diagnosed over a five year period. Approximately one-third of those tumours were missed by mammography and were found on palpation either by self-examination or by a doctor in the interval between two screenings. This group of tumours tended to be more aggressive and more invasive.[90]

Mammography's ability to find tumours is age-dependent, which also makes its use as a screening tool questionable, says oncologist Siddhartha Mukherjee. He notes that women over fifty have an increased incidence of breast cancer, so more tumours will be diagnosed by any means, including mammography.[91] In contrast, women under fifty have fewer malignant tumours, and, therefore, those tumours picked up tend to include more false positives.

Finally, renowned author Samuel Epstein reports that the routine practice of taking two films for each breast annually in premenopausal women results in an exposure to radiation that is 500 times the dose from a single chest X-ray. He comments that this is 25 times higher than the Environmental Protection Agency's recommended dosage of whole body radiation from local nuclear industries. This amount of radiation increases the risk of breast cancer by more than 1 percent annually. As there is a cumulative effect, ten years of mammography screening will increase the breast cancer risk by 10 percent in premenopausal women. Those women who are silent carriers of certain genes that increase their risk of breast cancer may account for 20 percent of breast cancer diagnoses annually in the US, especially

90 Gladwell, M. (2004, December 13). The picture problem: Mammography, air power and the limits of looking. *The New Yorker*. Retrieved from https://www.newyorker.com/magazine/2004/12/13/the-picture-problem.

91 Mukherjee, S. (2011). *The emperor of all maladies: A biography of cancer*. New York, NY: Scribner, p. 302.

those women under forty.[92] In women with a genetic predisposition for breast cancer (for example, with BRCA 1 or 2 or others), the risks of radiation from mammography can outweigh the benefits.[93]

In sum, factors such as overdiagnosis, subsequent overtreatment of benign lesions, the inability to pick up some small tumours, and the squeezing, traumatizing, and irradiating of the breast may all be reasons for some women to reconsider screening mammography. As Welch points out, at the very least, the question that a woman might ask about the utility of screening mammography has "more than one answer."[94] Since any benefits that mammography screening may offer must be weighed against the risks of this procedure, women should be informed about all implications of mammography screening so that they can make an informed choice.

Despite evidence that mammograms are of limited use as a screening tool for detecting early breast cancer, they are a major source of profit for the medical industry. This may be a factor driving their overuse. In the province of Ontario, government-generated financial incentives for doctors may contribute to their bias in favour of suggesting mammography screening to their patients. A conversation between doctor and patient on risks and benefits can take the same amount of time as a referral for a mammogram, but may be less financially lucrative. The Ontario government pays doctors a $2,200 bonus

92   Epstein, S. (2010, October 15). Breast cancer unawareness month: Rethinking mammograms. *Huffpost Life*. Retrieved from https://www.huffingtonpost.com/samuel-s-epstein/the-breast-cancer-unaware_b_754641.html

93   Berrington de Gonzalez, A., Berg, C. D., Visvanathan, K., & Robson, M. (2009). Estimated risk of radiation induced breast cancer from mammographic screening for young BRCA mutation carriers. *Journal of the National Cancer Institute, 101*(3), 205-209. https://doi.org/10.1093/jnci/djn440

94   Bleyer, A., & Welch, H. G. (2012). Effects of three decades of screening mammography on breast cancer incidence. *New England Journal of Medicine, 367*, 1998-2005. https://doi.org/10.1056/NEJMoa1206809

per year if 75 percent of their eligible patients are referred for routine mammography. Since having the conversation may be a less attractive option, patients may be ill informed about the limited benefits of mammography screening along with the associated risks.[95]

There has been a one-third reduction in mortality since screening mammography began, but this could also be attributed to improved therapies rather than to mammography. These improved therapies include hormonal interventions that work by suppressing the production of estrogen (excess estrogen feeds breast cancer).[96] Tamoxifen, aromatase inhibitors, and removal of ovaries can all reduce breast cancer mortality no matter the size of the tumour. Other natural and alternative methods to manage estrogen overload include, but are not limited to, Myomins, which have no side effects and have been found to shrink tumours in some studies; a diet that includes flax seeds, fermented foods such as miso, and turmeric; and exercise.

MRI

MRI is approximately 90 percent sensitive in picking up things that should be checked further. However, some studies note that its accuracy (specificity) in identifying cancer amongst these findings, rather than a benign finding, is no better than mammograms.[97,98] Moreover,

95   Glauser, W., Taylor, M., & Nolan, M. (2015, April 23). Are breast cancer screening programs justified? *Healthy Debate*. Retrieved from https://healthydebate.ca/2015/04/topic/breast-cancer-screening-justified

96   Welch, H. G., Prorok, P. C., O'Malley, A. J., & Kramer, B. S. (2016). Breast-cancer tumor size, overdiagnosis, and mammography screening effectiveness. *New England Journal of Medicine, 375*(15), 1438-1447. https://doi.org/10.1056/NEJMoa1600249

97   Saputo, L. (2003). *Beyond Mammography*. Walnut Creek, CA: Health Medicine Center. Retrieved from http://www.imageofgoodhealth.com/wp-content/uploads/2011/11/beyondmamm.pdf

98   Friedrich, M. (1998). MRI of the breast: State of the art. *European Radiology, 8*(5), 707-725. https://doi.org/10.1007/s003300050463

it is unclear what detrimental effects may come from exposure to the MRI's magnetic fields. Additionally, the contrast dye, gadolinium, that many institutions insist on using when doing breast MRIs is a neurotoxin. There is some evidence that it remains in the body and is released into tissue, rather than eliminated, as originally thought.[99]

Thermograms

Breast thermography is an accurate and sensitive procedure and a great alternative to screening mammography for young women who might otherwise suffer negative consequences from years of mammography and radiation exposure. Cancer cells divide rapidly and require increased blood flow, which in turn generates increased heat. This process of thermovascular change is picked up by thermograms. These tools serve as a safe, early warning system, flagging changes in the breast 8-10 years before other detection methods. Thermography is also a safe way to obtain baseline readings early on in a woman's life.[100] Studies that compared the effectiveness of mammography, clinical exam, and thermography found thermography increased the diagnostic accuracy of the first two technologies to between 85% and 98%.[101]

Mastectomies

The climate of fear amongst women induced by overdiagnosis and misdiagnosis has also led to a surge in demand for mastectomies, a

---

99   Rogosnitzky, M., & Branch, S. (2016). Gadolinium-based contrast agent toxicity: A review of known and proposed mechanisms. *Biometals, 29*(3), 365-76. https://doi.org/10.1007/s10534-016-9931-7

100   Saputo, L. (2003). *Beyond Mammography.* Walnut Creek, CA: Health Medicine Center. Retrieved from http://www.imageofgoodhealth.com/wp-content/uploads/2011/11/beyondmamm.pdf

101   Amalu, W. C. (2003). Review of breast thermography. *International Academy of Clinical Thermography.* Retrieved from http://www.breastthermography.com/infrared_imaging_review.htm

throwback to the sixties. In the late sixties and early seventies, women became more vocal about their medical needs. At that time, routine radical mastectomies were re-evaluated as women increasingly refused these disfiguring procedures.[102,103] The story of oncologist Vera Peters is retold by radiation oncologist and playwright Charles Hayter earlier in this book. Peters successfully lobbied in Canada for women to forego radical mastectomies in favour of lumpectomies, which her research indicated was equally effective in many cases. Many of Peters' findings were echoed in the eighties in the United States by University of Pennsylvania oncologist and researcher, Bernard Fisher. His work, which included applying the first clinical trials and statistical methodology to breast cancer research, was considered pioneering. It resulted in overturning the routinely performed radical and disfiguring mastectomy in favour of less extensive localized surgery. At that time, he faced much criticism for claiming that lumpectomy was as effective as mastectomy in treating some breast cancers. He believed cancer to be a systemic disease and that women who had radical mastectomies did not acquire any benefits related to survival, recurrence, or mortality.[104] In retrospect, viewing cancer as a systemic problem was a progressive notion and aligned him with the more alternative and holistically oriented practitioners today who feel cancer needs to be managed as a whole body issue.

102 Lerner, B. (2001). No shrinking violet: Rose Kushner and the rise of American breast cancer activism. *Western Journal Medicine, 174*(5), 362-365. Retrieved from https://www.ncbi.nlm.nih.gov/pmc/articles/PMC1071404/

103 Mukherjee, S. (2011). *The emperor of all maladies: A biography of cancer.* New York, NY: Scribner, p. 199.

104 Fisher, B., Redmond, C., Poisson, R., & Margolese, R. (1989). Eight-year results of a randomized clinical trial comparing total mastectomy and lumpectomy with or without irradiation in the treatment of breast cancer. *New England Journal of Medicine, 320*, 822-828. https://doi.org/10.1056/NEJM198903303201302

Despite the pioneering work of these two doctors and the change they effected in the practice of radical mastectomy, there has been a recent swing back to this radical and disfiguring procedure. The increase in findings of DCIS since screening mammography was put in place has generated a surge in mastectomies. Yet this radical procedure may not provide a significant benefit in many cases of DCIS, and may bring with it pain, disfigurement, and debilitation as described above. In a large study of prophylactic mastectomy, Todd Tuttle, surgical oncologist at the University of Minnesota and colleagues, reported a 180 percent jump between 1998 and 2005 among women given a new diagnosis of DCIS in one breast who opted to have both breasts removed prophylactically. The mortality rate over a ten-year period for women with this diagnosis is 2 percent, so the benefits seem of small value.[105]

Between 1998 and 2011, the rates of bilateral mastectomy for women in the U.S. with various types of breast cancer (who were candidates for lumpectomy) rose from 2 percent to 12.3 percent.[106] Despite this surge, some studies have indicated that mastectomy will not prevent metastasis and that the survival benefits are negligible. Contralateral prophylactic mastectomy is a procedure where the healthy breast is removed along with the breast that has cancer. This decision is made by some in an effort to prevent breast cancer from returning at a later time in the unaffected breast. However, various studies have

105 Tuttle, T. M., Jarosek, S., Habermann, E. B., Arrington, A., Abraham, A., Morris, T. J., & Virnig, B. A. (2009). Increasing rates of contralateral prophylactic mastectomy among patients with ductal carcinoma in situ. *Journal of Clinical Oncology, 27*(9), 1362-1367. https://doi.org/10.1200/JCO.2008.20.1681

106 Wise, J. (2016). Rates of prophylactic mastectomy triple in decade. *British Medical Journal, 2016,* 352. https://doi.org/10.1136/bmj.i1504

reported a negligible survival benefit for this procedure.[107,108,109] Dr. Ann Partridge reports that removing a woman's healthy breast offers no survival benefit. If cancer does return, she notes, it is usually not to the other breast.[110]

> Dr. Ann Partridge is Associate Professor at Harvard Medical School, Co-Founder and Director of Young and Strong Program for Young Women with Breast Cancer and Director Dana-Farber Adult Survivorship Program.

Given the very small risk of breast cancer developing in the other breast later among women who have cancer in one breast, systemic therapy (that is, hormonally targeted therapy to suppress estrogen overload) is one possible alternative to prophylactic mastectomy. It

107   Portschy, P. R., Kuntz, K. M., Tuttle, T. M. (2014). Survival outcomes after contralateral prophylactic mastectomy: A decision analysis. *Journal of National Cancer Institute, 106*(8). https://doi.org/10.1093/jnci/dju160

108   Kurian, A. W., Lichtensztain, D. Y., Keegan, T. H., Nelson, D. O., Clarke, C. A., & Gomez, S. L. (2014). Use of and mortality after bilateral mastectomy compared with other surgical treatments for breast cancer in California. *Journal of American Medical Association, 312*(9), 902-914. https://doi.org/10.1001/jama.2014.10707

109   Wong, S. M., Freedman, R. A., Sagara, Y., Aydogan, F., Barry, W. T., & Golshan, M. (2017). Growing use of contralateral prophylactic mastectomy despite no improvement in long-term survival for invasive breast cancer. *Annals of Surgery, 265*(3), 581-589. https://doi.org/10.1097/SLA.0000000000001698

110   Partridge, A. (2015, February 24). Now that I have breast cancer on one side, should I remove both breasts? *Susan G. Komen*. Retrieved from https://ww5.komen.org/Blog/Now-that-I-have-breast-cancer-on-one-side,-should-I-remove-both-breasts-/

can lower the risk of recurrence in those women who can benefit from an estrogen suppressing treatment.[111]

Radiation

Radiation has long-lasting effects. I discovered this fact by accident in 2014, some years after my own treatment had ended, while reading a local newspaper. The article recounted extensive stories on the long-term effects of radiation for breast cancer that is targeted near the heart. Cardiac exposure in chest radiation can result in scarring, stiffened heart muscles, and narrowed valves and vessels, producing coronary heart disease years, sometimes decades, later. While not everyone irradiated near the heart develops these problems, it is considered a bigger risk factor for cancer patients who received radiation prior to 2002, when doses were less targeted. A 2013 study published in the New England Journal of Medicine looked at 2,168 women who had radiation for breast cancer between 1958 and 2001. In this study, each unit of radiation, known as a "gray" that the heart was exposed to, increased the rate of a major coronary event by 7.4 percent.[112]

Radiation, though employed in an attempt to destroy cancer, is itself carcinogenic. The frightening effects of radiation exposure were graphically related in a story by Veronique Greenwood, a journalist and relative of an employee at the Marie Curie Radium Institute in Paris.[113] In this article, she describes how Marie Curie, who was fascinated by both the destructive and regenerative effects of radium,

111 Gretchen, L. G., Curtis, R. E., Pfeiffer, R. M., Mullooly, M., Ntowe, E. A., Hoover, R. N., ... Berrington de Gonzalez, A. (2017). Adjuvant endocrine therapy and risk of contralateral breast cancer among U.S. women with breast cancer. *Journal of American Medical Association Oncology, 3*(2), 186-193. https://doi.org/10.1001/jamaoncol.2016.3340

112 White, N. J. (2014, January 25). Breathing technique helps protect heart from radiation. *The Toronto Star*, p. L8.

113 Greenwood, V. (2014, December 3). My great-great-aunt discovered francium. And it killed her. *New York Times Magazine*, pp. 52-56.

achieved celebrity status as a result of her pioneering work on radio-active substances. Greenwood reminds us, however, that alpha and beta particles emitted in radiation attack DNA and that the mutations they cause can lead to cancer. Radioactive elements that are absorbed in the body can concentrate in the bones, where they continue their decay, in effect poisoning someone for as long as that person lives. This was indeed the case for many employees of the Radium Institute, including Curie herself, as they and she succumbed to painful and disfiguring illnesses and death from radiation-related cancers.

In relation to breast cancer, some studies say radiation does not increase your chance of surviving the illness because it targets only the localized cancer in the breast. According to Naturopaths Steve Austin and Cathy Hitchcock in their well-researched book, "*Breast Cancer: What You Should Know (But May Not Be Told) about Prevention, Diagnosis, and Treatment,* "distal metastasis, which is the spread of cancer beyond the breast, is what kills the patient, and this is unaffected by radiating the breast tumor.[114] In short, the area that is radiated after surgery in the breast area targets a local recurrence only, while predisposing you to collateral damage, which can include other cancers later. In fact, not only does it not protect against metastasis, but when radiation is used in cases of DCIS, often referred to as stage "0" cancer, it can contribute to mortality if it is administered on the same side as the heart.[115] Scandinavian researchers have examined whether treatment of stage 1 breast cancer with surgery alone can reduce the local recurrence rate to an acceptable level without

---

Retrieved from https://www.nytimes.com/2014/12/07/magazine/my-great-great-aunt-discovered-francium-and-it-killed-her.html

114 Austin, S., & Hitchcock, C. (1994). *Breast cancer: What you should know (but may not be told) about prevention, diagnosis, and treatment.* Rocklin, CA: Prima, p. 58.

115 Esserman, L., & Yau, C. (2015). Rethinking the standard for ductal carcinoma in situ treatment. *Journal of the American Medical Association Oncology, 1*(7), 881-883. https://doi.org/10.1001/jamaoncol.2015.2607

radiation in a number of studies. They found that the two treatment groups (radiation and no-radiation) did not differ in overall survival when examined over a 20 year period. The data indicated that radiation given routinely in cases where the tumour can be considered controlled by surgery alone constitutes overtreatment in 80 percent of patients. A group of Swedish researchers studied lumpectomy in women with an invasive breast cancer, which had not spread to their nodes and with tumours that were less than two centimetres. They found that after five years, almost nine out of ten women had not suffered a local recurrence. At the ten-year mark post-diagnosis for those who had radiation, there was a 16 percent reduction in local recurrence, compared with those who did not have radiation after surgery. However, radiation after surgery did not reduce distant recurrences or improve survival.[116,117] This data is important to consider when weighing the benefits of radiation against its long-term risks, which could include other cancers and damage to the heart or lungs.

Chemotherapy

In an effort to wipe out cancer at all costs, massive infusions of cash were made and aggressive multi-institute drug trials were put in place at various times over the last fifty years. Despite this, little progress in curing cancer was made, according to Oncologist Siddhartha Mukherjee in his book "The Emperor of All Maladies: A Biography of Cancer." He notes that the midpoint of the most aggressive expansion of chemo occurred between

116 Wickberg, A., Holmberg, L., Adami, H-O., Magnuson, A., Villman, K., & Liljegren, G. (2014). Sector resection with or without post-operative radiotherapy for stage I breast cancer: 20-year results of a randomized trial. *Journal of Clinical Oncology, 32*(8), 791-797. https://doi.org/10.1200/JCO.2013.50.6600

117 Cohen, A., Ljunggvist, U., Tabár, L., Bergkvist, L., Johannson, L.,Holmberg, L., ... Graffman, S. (1990). Sector resection with or without post-operative radiotherapy for stage I breast cancer: A randomized trial. *Journal of the National Cancer Institute, 82*(4), 277-282. Retrieved from https://www.ncbi.nlm.nih.gov/pubmed/2405171

1984 and 1985, when nearly six thousand articles were published on chemotherapy in medical journals. However, no new strategies were developed for curing solid malignant tumours (such as breast, lung and colon) that were in an advanced stage ,with chemotherapy alone. Many of the brutal drug trials compromised the quality of life of cancer patients, maybe only prolonging their life by a few months while simultaneously causing terrible side effects, sometimes even contributing to their early death. For instance, Adriamycin, a drug which is still widely used today, could cause serious damage to the heart. Despite these enormous efforts to wipe out cancer, Mukherjee reports that by the end of the 1990s, screening tests did not improve outcome, cancer was still elusive, and doctors continued to administer radical treatments without understanding the cancer cell. He writes that by 2004, doctors were still struggling to deal with the fact that some cancer cells carrying mutated genes could survive a chemo barrage, and then migrate to other parts of the body where they formed metastasis. Doctors remain uncertain as to which of those cells will behave this way. Moreover, because chemotherapy targets cellular growth, it also attacks normal growth as well as uncontrolled growth hence its collateral cost.[118] In a recent article in the New York Times Magazine, Mukherjee describes a shift in the last decade in the treatment of certain cancers. While most cancer patients are still treated with the standardized protocols, he notes that some people with difficult to treat cancers who relapse are receiving more individualized treatments. There are signals of a shift in the stance of some oncologists. While previously they may have been terrified not to follow strict patient protocols, some are now open to more flexible treatment approaches that allow for creative interventions that are unique to a particular individual's cancer.[119]

According to research published in the New England Journal of Medicine, many women undergo chemotherapy to lower their chances

118 Mukherjee, S. (2011). *The emperor of all maladies: A biography of cancer*. New York, NY: Scribner, pp. 206-208, 304, 403-407.

119 Mukherjee, S. (2016, May 15). The new anatomy of cancer. *The New York Times Magazine*. Retrieved from https://www.nytimes.com/2016/05/15/magazine/oncologist-improvisation.html

of the cancer recurring. Nevertheless, for a vast majority of women, the cancer will not recur, with or without chemotherapy, and the chemotherapy will only help a fraction of those treated with it. Because doctors cannot tell with certainty which women fall into this category many women who do not need chemotherapy will receive it.[120] Statistics related to benefits for chemotherapy have ranged from only a two percent benefit in five and ten year survival in the United States, to a seven to eleven percent benefit in younger women under the age of fifty. However, the collateral damage of this intervention may include ovarian failure with resultant infertility, sexual dysfunction, hair loss, bone loss, weight gain, neurocognitive changes, cardiac toxicity, and secondary malignancy.[121] Given such a paltry yield, and the toxicity and collateral damage these drugs inflict, these results indicate that this might be an intervention worth questioning. Moreover, cancer cells frequently mutate and become smarter at neutralizing even aggressive cocktails. Gene expression tests such as MammaPrint and Oncotype DX have been developed and used more recently in certain patients to help determine whether they are at low risk of metastasis and can safely skip chemotherapy. At the time of completing this book, the New England Journal of Medicine published results of a nine year study comparing outcomes in 10,000 women with early stage breast cancers who were treated with or without chemotherapy following surgery. The study employed the predictive results of Oncotype DX test in determining risk. Researchers found that chemotherapy was unnecessary in about 83 percent of women with early stage breast cancer. This includes cases where the cancer had not spread to the nodes under the arm, was positive for estrogen or progesterone, and HER 2 negative. They

120   Pollack, A. (2004, December 11). Data mounts on avoiding chemotherapy. *The New York Times Magazine* Retrieved from https://www.nytimes.com/2004/12/11/health/data-mounts-on-avoiding-chemotherapy.html

121   Mayer, E. L. (2013). Early and late long-term effects of adjuvant chemotherapy. *American Society Clinical Oncology Education Book, 2013,* 9-14. https://doi.org/10.1200/EdBook_AM.2013.33.9

concluded that chemotherapy offered no additional treatment benefit for this group of women.[122]

> HER 2 positive breast cancer: a breast cancer that occurs in approximately one in five breast cancers. A genetic mutation causes an excess of a protein called human epidermal growth factor receptor 2, which results in growth of cancer cells. Herceptin, a medication which has been approved in Canada since 2005, has significantly increased survival in women with this particular cancer.

In a TED Talk given in October 2009, Dr. David Agus challenged the use of many conventional chemotherapies.[123] He cited an important study of 1,800 women with premenopausal breast cancer that was reported on in the New England Journal of Medicine in February 2009.[124] This study found that a bone density drug called zoledronic acid given to women with early stage breast cancer in addition to hormone suppressant treatment reduced new primary cancers by 30 percent and reduced recurrence of their cancers by 35 percent. Agus claimed that most chemo drugs have not been shown to touch cancer cells and that they may instead be disrupting a complex system, a task that can perhaps be performed by less toxic drugs.

---

122 Sparano, J., Gray, R. J., Makower, D. F., & Pritchard, K. I. (2018). Adjuvant chemotherapy guided by a 21-gene expression assay in breast cancer. *New England Journal of Medicine, 379*, 111-121. https://doi.org/10.1056/NEJMoa1804710

123 Agus, D. [TED Med]. (2009). A new strategy in the war on cancer [Video file]. Retrieved from https://www.ted.com/talks/david_agus_a_new_strategy_in_the_war_on_cancer/up-next

124 Gnant, M., Mlineritsch, B., Schippinger, W., Luschin-Ebengreuth, G., Pöstlberger, S., Menzel, C., … Greil, R. (2009). Endocrine therapy plus Zoledronic acid in premenopausal breast cancer. *New England Journal of Medicine, 360*, 679-691. https://doi.org/10.1056/NEJMoa0806285

Dr. David Agus is an oncologist and professor of medicine at the University of Southern California, author of *The End of Illness*, and CBS news contributor.

The journalist Rose Kushner, a renowned advocate for change in the field of breast cancer in the seventies and eighties, and the first lay member of the National Cancer Advisory Board in the US, captured what many women feel about the horrors of chemotherapy.[125] Kushner cited the almost cavalier attitude of the medical community to this treatment at times. She noted that side effects are often minimized. And while sometimes life-threatening side effects may be considered tolerable or acceptable, others such as vomiting so hard that you break the blood vessels in your eyes or going bald do not even warrant a mention. She herself refused chemo when first diagnosed, believing it to be excessive treatment. Too often, I have personally witnessed or heard second-hand a mirroring of Kushner's description of the medical reaction, or lack of it, in relation to the side effects from chemo. Only a few years ago, a friend of mine who had been treated for breast cancer at a major Toronto hospital related her oncologist's philosophy, which was to "throw everything at her breast cancer except the kitchen sink." Despite the barrage she endured to beat the cancer, she died only a few years later. Another friend of mine with breast cancer recalled foam coming out of her eyes and multiple teeth cracking during chemo, complaints that were dismissed by her doctors as bearing no relationship to the treatment.

Given the studies and data and the collateral damage these drugs may have, women should be informed of the very limited and uncertain beneficial effects of some of these therapies so they can make more informed choices. Additionally, knowing in advance about alternatives that can minimize collateral damage is crucial.

---

125 Kushner, R. (1984). Is aggressive adjuvant chemotherapy the Halsted radical of the '80s? *CA: A Cancer Journal for Clinicians, 34*(6), 345-351. https://doi.org/10.3322/canjclin.34.6.345

CHAPTER 14

My Story: Reflections

My tumour was early stage with no nodal involvement and moderately differentiated, a term which indicates the degree to which it resembles a normal cell. On a scale of 1 to 3, it was considered the most aggressive "grade." The four rounds of chemotherapy and five weeks of radiation after surgery that I opted for were, I now believe, unnecessary given the questionable gains these treatments offer and the collateral damage they inflict.

Cancer indicates your immune system is not strong enough to override cancer cells. Further decimating it, as with chemotherapy, does not make sense to me. Like most women, when I received a diagnosis of breast cancer, I was ill-informed about the many possible interventions from across the spectrum to treat and manage it. (These include many of the treatments discussed earlier in this book.) Fear and ignorance propelled me to act quickly and follow a conventional path that included surgery, chemotherapy, radiation and hormonal treatments. Though I was told I would feel fine six months to two years after treatment with chemotherapy and radiation, it took me four years and many alternative interventions to regain my strength.

I was diagnosed with breast cancer one year after my marriage suddenly ended. I found myself in a bleak state, a place where I could find little meaning in my life. No doubt my immune system was severely weakened by my sense of meaninglessness at this time. I believe that this trauma and the subsequent psychological fallout along with any predisposing factors I may have had pushed me over the edge, resulting in my disease. I was fortunate enough during the treatment to become involved with a wonderful, caring partner who helped to extricate me from the black hole I was in. The feelings this relationship generated, helped my body to muster more forces to fight the cancer.

My experience with chemotherapy and suffering the consequences is the single most important factor in my writing this book. Going through chemotherapy places a cancer diagnosis in a different and more serious light. At times during this treatment I felt like an empty shell, sapped of all strength, enthusiasm, and hope. I lived from moment to moment with little sense of a future. I suspect these feelings are familiar to anyone who has endured this treatment. Dealing with both the experience and the fallout from the treatment left me with a determination to do anything I could to prevent a recurrence.

It has been my observation that those women who do not have chemotherapy, but perhaps only surgery, or surgery and radiation, often take the prospect of a recurrence less seriously. A wish to prevent a recurrence sent me down a path of exploration to determine other, gentler remedies to shore up my immune system and to inform myself about other interventions in case of recurrence. This book also grew out of my need to regain a feeling of control over my health. Writing for me has always been a way to lend meaning when I've found myself in a dark place. As I began to write about my marriage breakdown and my new relationship in the context of the diagnosis, I began to feel better. But I had a real health problem, and though I was assured I'd feel well soon after the treatments ended, I felt weak, depressed, and pessimistic about the future. I needed to look elsewhere to regain a sense of robustness and some of the control the cancer had robbed me of.

The more information I gathered, the more this book took hold. One practitioner I spoke with opened a door to another, showing me a new, hopeful path that would ultimately lead to the sense of well-being and health I now enjoy. Reassuring faces that I met along the way, such as those of Alvin Pettle and Sat Dharam Kaur, who believe in their interventions as preventive measures, helped me to see I had a future.

The lingering feelings of debilitation sent me on a search for remedies to undo the ravages of the chemotherapy and radiation. I found those remedies in the integrative and alternative world. Ten years post-diagnosis, I continue to come across information that would have helped me to make more informed and, ultimately, better choices about the path I wished to follow. My personal experience and subsequent research over these last few years have led me to believe that relying solely on conventional interventions, such as surgery, chemotherapy, radiation, and standard of care hormonal treatments, may not be sufficient or even necessary. Other interventions from across the health care spectrum, that consider and include integrative and alternative solutions, should be considered in managing a cancer diagnosis.

I believe that my recovery so far has occurred in spite of the chemo, not because of it. That is, had I not so determinedly followed an alternative path to health after completing my conventional treatment, I might not have achieved the recovery I now enjoy. At the very least, conventional treatment, if that is the route you choose, is merely a start, in my opinion, and aiding your body in strengthening its immune system is imperative after the barrage it sustains from both the cancer and the treatments. On a personal and intuitive level, it's hard for me to believe that anything that almost wipes out your immune system, which is the case with many chemotherapies, could be curative. Chemotherapy compromises the immune system over the long term, predisposing one to other illnesses, including cancers. It is my belief that for too many people, chemo is more destructive than beneficial, and that the damage it does is far reaching and counterproductive. Whether or not you do the chemo, uncertainty remains, and there are no guarantees. I do not believe that chemotherapy is an "insurance policy" against recurrence, as friends and doctors suggested prior to my choice to do this treatment.

As some of the professionals in this book highlight, the body needs help to stimulate its own defence system to fight cancer and alter the environment in which the cancer thrived in the first place. Non-toxic alternative remedies can aid in this process, sustaining any gains and improving prognosis. During my own chemotherapy, I stopped taking important antioxidant supplements because my oncologist said they might interfere with the effects of the chemo. For instance, she advised me against using vitamin C, though many believe it can protect normal cells and speed up recovery. In retrospect, I feel not using this important vitamin was the wrong move and that continuing with it at that time might have hastened my recovery.

Regarding radiation, the immediate symptom from treatment is merely fatigue, but radiation itself sits in one's bones for life, possibly triggering another cancer later. Moreover, many studies suggest there is no difference in life expectancy with or without radiation when the breast cancer tumour is small, since radiation deals only with a local recurrence, not a distant one.

In my attempts to manage the genetic predisposition I may have for cancer, I employ various interventions that serve as preventive measures. I am more meticulous about my diet, which is, as much as possible, sugar-free, carbohydrate-free, and mostly dairy-free (except for kefir, which acts as an important probiotic). This also keeps my body in a more alkaline state. Sugar and white flour may contribute to inflammatory processes in the body, and sugar may feed cancer. When I was going through chemo and lost a lot of weight, I asked about eating sugar-laden chocolate. A well-meaning nurse responded with, "You can eat what you like." Given what I now know about sugar and cancer, this comment horrifies me. I recently stumbled upon an article in the New York Times Magazine in which the oncologist Siddhartha Mukherjee calls for a long overdue 'careful scientific examination of diet as medicine' in the field of oncology.[126] He confirms my belief

---

126 Mukherjee, S. (2018, December 9). It's time to study whether eating particular diets can help heal us. *The New York Times Magazine*. Retrieved from https://www.nytimes.com/2018/12/05/magazine/its-time-to-study-whether-eating-particular-diets-can-help-heal-us.html

and that of many professionals in this book that diet may have an important impact on health..

I continue to take daily supplements of compounded C0Q10 with B6, B12, folic acid, indole-3-carbinol, and vitamin D3. When cooking, I add turmeric powder to as many things as possible. I add pepper as well to ensure absorption of the turmeric through the stomach wall. I balance my estrogen using Myomins, a supplement which generally has no side effects and helps the liver rid itself of toxins including excess estrone and estradiol (components of estrogen). Daily sublingual DHEA drops under the tongue monitored with regular blood tests bring my cortisol levels down, and transvaginal estriol, that is estriol cream applied inside the vagina, bumps up the ratio of the good hormones. I try to improve the quality of my sleep with 20 milligrams of melatonin nightly, which rolls back my biological clock and boosts my immune system.

One of the first things I did after finishing treatment, on the urging of my naturopath, was to attend to my mouth health. I had all amalgam in my mouth removed by a holistic dentist who used equipment that prevented vapours being inhaled into my lungs during the extraction process. Amalgam emits gas for life and, therefore, it is believed by some, compromises health indefinitely. I had one root canal forty years ago, and I struggle with how to deal with this. I have decided for now to leave it, since it was done in the seventies and may have silver pins, not toxic metal ones. Should I need another root canal in the future, I would opt to have the tooth removed and would seriously consider a zirconium implant, which is the newest generation of biocompatible implants. For other dental problems, I always insist on non-toxic solutions. For instance, recently my dentist employed a polycarboxylate cement, which is BPA-free, in completing a crown. Most importantly, I have learned to raise my concerns and to question standard solutions.

Another intervention that I regard as very important for my post-treatment recovery is acupuncture. It helped me to overcome the extreme fatigue I felt by opening up blocked meridians, which cause a damming up of toxins. There is some evidence that acupuncture augments our immune response by stimulating NK (natural killer) cells and that it can also reduce tumour size.[127] I can't praise acupuncture enough, as it came to my rescue when doctors responded with bafflement to my physical complaints. I continue to use acupuncture now and then to maintain my well-being or attend to particular complaints.

We are all subjected to radiation from a multitude of sources in our environment, but it is possible to avoid some of it, especially the radiation in some forms of breast cancer prevention, such as mammograms. I personally refuse routine mammograms. I worry about the intense squeezing that can break capillaries which some say can spread malignant cells around the body. Additionally, mammograms can easily miss tumours in dense breasts.[128] Studies such as the Canadian study by Narod et al., which was mentioned earlier in this book, also suggest mammography screening makes no difference to mortality in breast cancer. My breast cancer was found on palpation by a doctor one week after a negative mammogram result. I was personally encouraged to have mammography from the age of thirty-five, given that my mother had breast cancer when she was sixty-one. I wonder about the damage from years of mammograms and concurrent radiation. Of the many doctors I had in Canada, the US, and Norway over a period of nearly thirty years, not one ever discussed the contraindications with me. Since surgery for breast cancer in my fifties and after learning more about the very limited diagnostic ability of mammography, the hazards related to the squeezing, radiation, and the possibility of cancer overdiagnosis using this instrument, I have

---

127 Frączek, P., Kilan-Kita, A., Püsküllüoglu, M., & Krzemieniecki, K. Acupuncture as anticancer treatment? *Contemporary Oncology*, *20*(6), 453-457. https://doi.org/10.5114/wo.2016.65604

128 Pisano, E. D., Hendrick, R. E., Yaffe, M. J., Baum, J. K., Acharyya, S., Cormack, J. B., ... Gatsonis, C. A. (2008). Diagnostic accuracy of digital versus film mammography: Exploratory analysis of selected population subgroups in DMIST. *Radiology*, *246*(2). https://10.1148/radiol.2461070200

now personally decided not to have further screening mammograms. I will have a mammogram only if it is absolutely necessary to confirm or rule out a questionable result from another diagnostic tool, that is, for the purposes of diagnosis, not screening. Instead, I have annual ultrasound exams that can detect whether a lump is hollow and fluid-filled or hard, although not whether it is malignant. This instrument is safe and non-invasive. I also have annual thermograms, which determine whether there is an inflammatory process underway based on heat appearing on an infrared picture, and I undergo periodic MRIs. MRI scanners are sensitive instruments, and their use may expose one to possible overdiagnosis, but MRIs offer information that the other technologies do not. Finally, my oncology surgeon physically examines my breast annually, which reassures me more than any machinery.

If I could go back in time, empowered by my current knowledge, I would make different choices at the time of diagnosis. I would not succumb to the pressure I felt to act swiftly, but would take my time to examine alternatives that are less invasive and destructive than those I opted for. Cancer takes years to appear, and giving yourself time to research options and make choices you feel comfortable with, may afford you a better outcome. I personally would not do conventional chemo or radiation, but would employ a multi-pronged approach along with surgery, which I would carefully time. I would seek out treatments that would boost my immune system.

Nowadays, when I feel a twinge or ache in my body, my fears resurface, and when that twinge vanishes, my fears dissipate. Recently, I had a squamous cell skin cancer on my arm. Hearing the word "cancer" set off a cascade of worries about the state of my immune system, although this particular skin cancer is usually non-invasive and is very treatable. My integrative doctor noticed that my C-reactive protein levels did not indicate any signs of inflammation in my body, suggesting this was a localized cancer. This result was reassuring, but the diagnosis suggested I needed to be more vigilant. It was a reminder that cancer lurks around the corner, and rather than being cured with surgery, chemotherapy, and radiation, it is an ongoing management issue.

We need to transform the hand we are dealt, employing interventions that make sense to us, some of which have been highlighted in this book. In an effort to take responsibility for my own health, I myself have followed many practices described here and found relief in doing so. Along the way I was lucky enough to have met many supportive and empathic professionals who helped me on my journey. I don't know what my future holds, but thanks to all my discoveries, I now enjoy a sense of physical well-being that was hard to imagine eleven years ago when I finished chemotherapy and radiation treatment.

CHAPTER 15

Conclusions

Breast cancer mortality has dropped about **28%** in the last three decades, and certain treatments have improved, but many uncertainties in both treating and curing cancer remain.[129] Unable to keep up with rapidly changing scientific data, doctors may fall back on the tried and true standard protocols that often paint cancer treatment from one patient to the next with the same brush. However, the difficulty with the "one size fits all" cancer therapy approach is that the disease is imagined as mostly uniform based on its location in the body. Yet the reality is that, once a tumour is formed, each one "behaves" and "moves" differently, Mukherjee notes.[130] Moreover, even very aggressive cocktails may be of little use because cancer cells easily mutate, and even neutralize drugs, rendering the chemo useless.

Facts like these have brought us all to what Mukherjee calls the "mapless moment." Doctors and researchers have become more

---

129 Bleyer, A., & Welch, H. G. (2012). Effects of three decades of screening mammography on breast cancer incidence, *New England Journal of Medicine, 367*, 1998-2005. https://doi.org/10.1056/NEJMoa1206809

130 Mukherjee, S. (2016, May 12). The new anatomy of cancer. *The New York Times Magazine*. Retrieved from https://www.nytimes.com/2016/05/15/magazine/oncologist-improvisation.html?mtrref=undefined

curious about the particular personality of each individual cancer and the necessity of understanding that in order to adequately treat it.[131] Therapies that target abnormalities have improved survival with some cancers, however, not all cells that mutate will cause cancer. Targeting all mutations could do a lot of damage to harmless cells. Breast cancer involves fifty to eighty genetic mutations, making a targeted treatment very complex and overwhelming.[132]

Immunotherapy, hailed as one of the new frontiers in cancer research, employs the body's own immune system in fighting cancer. However, it can cause severe life-threatening side effects in up to 54 percent of patients who are treated with these drugs, making the collateral damage a huge factor to consider.[133] Dr. Robert Wachter, chairman of the Department of Medicine at the University of California, San Francisco writes that only about 15 percent of patients with advanced cancer could benefit from immunotherapy. He adds that it's impossible to predict which patients will respond to this treatment.[134]

In a recent article in the New York Times Magazine, oncologist Siddhartha Mukherjee reflected on his experience running clinical trials that were testing new medicines to treat certain cancers. He points out that less than one percent of the several million chemical

131 Mukherjee, S. (2016, May 12). The new anatomy of cancer. *The New York Times Magazine*. Retrieved from https://www.nytimes.com/2016/05/15/magazine/oncologist-improvisation.html?mtrref=undefined

132 Mukherjee, S. (2010). *Emperor of all maladies: A biography of cancer*. New York, NY: Scriber, pp. 451-452.

133 Richtel, M. (2016, December 3). Immune system, unleashed by cancer therapy, can attack organs. *The New York Times Magazine*. Retrieved from https://www.nytimes.com/2016/12/03/health/immunotherapy-cancer.html

134 Wachter, R. W. (2018, April 18). The problem with miracle cancer cures. *The New York Times Magazine*. Retrieved from https://www.nytimes.com/2018/04/19/opinion/sunday/problem-miracle-cancer-cures.html

reactions in the human body are currently referred to in the medical pharmacopoeia, a fact that highlights the complexities of the human physiology. Cancer and its personality and behaviour are no exceptions, he says.[135]

All of these factors make the notion of a cure being found anytime soon elusive. Because overwhelming evidence indicates that there is little certainty regarding outcome with most cancers, doctors must remain flexible about treatment interventions and open to new ways of managing cancers that well-informed patients may present to them. More research and collaboration between conventional, integrative, and alternative practitioners is required. Research can lend credibility to interventions made by practitioners in the integrative and alternative world. Similarly, an openness to collaborative efforts across the spectrum can result in educating doctors as well as patients to the merits of interventions they may not be clear about. A multi-pronged approach in cancer management makes sense in light of these factors.

Patients must be clearly informed about the outcomes and collateral damage of current conventional treatments and be presented with all treatment options, including alternative ones. Patients who choose alternative or integrative treatments either adjunctively or in lieu of conventional treatments must be taken seriously by doctors, even if they feel ambivalent about patients straying from standard protocols. Cancer is a management issue, rather than something we can cure and forget about. Therefore, post-cancer bolstering of an already ailing immune system and keeping cancer cells, which we all have, in check makes eminent sense to me. David Servan-Schreiber, MD, renowned author of *Anticancer: A New Way of Life*, calls this "tending to the soil" in which the cancer grows to prevent further episodes. Dietary interventions, supplementation, hormonal balancing, exercise, acupuncture, minimization of chemical intake from our

135 Mukherjee, S. (2017, December 3). On medicine, a failure to heal. *The New York Times Magazine*. Retrieved from https://www.nytimes.com/2017/11/28/magazine/a-failure-to-heal.html

environment, tending to mouth health, and managing stress can be extremely helpful in this task.

I have learned in writing this book that there is not one single cure or intervention that alone will turn our medical fates around. Cancer has many causes and treatments that vary from one institution to the next and work differently on different people. There are many professionals who have their particular perspectives on keeping cancer at bay, and being apprised of these helps us to make informed and better decisions about how to proceed. Certainly, taking charge in this way has allowed me to put my experiences behind me much of the time, and to feel I have some control over a disease that might otherwise overwhelm me with its complexities and the uncertainties surrounding its management and prognosis.

If you are faced with this diagnosis, just remember that there are many practitioners around the world doing amazing things with cancer, and you need never feel that your options are limited to the harsh and relatively narrow range presented by conventional medicine. Seeking out these allies is part of the recovery, and you may find that making the journey will enhance your psychological and physical well-being.

ACKNOWLEDGEMENTS

I am very grateful to all the courageous practitioners and patients in this book who so generously shared their thoughts and time and who were a great inspiration to me. I am also immensely grateful to Malcolm Lester, retired publisher of Lester, Orpin and Denys for his unflagging support and encouragement throughout. He has always been available with thoughtful advice and feedback on all aspects of the book. His belief in the worth of this project helped to get it off the ground and to keep moving forward in the face of various setbacks. I am also so appreciative of Dr. Alvin Pettle, who was enormously helpful as a medical consultant on this book. He reinforced my belief that the information in this book must be shared, and his ongoing encouragement and interest were crucial forces in my sustaining the necessary momentum to complete this project. Thanks very much to Jenny Govier, editor, whose patience, skills and guidance were instrumental in this book taking shape, to Ali Cunliffe for her sharp journalistic editing skills, and generosity with her time and feedback, and to Cristina Khan whose promptness and acute editing skills were much appreciated. The many discussions with Dr. Ali Farahani, and Dr. Dana Colson about the relationship between illness and mouth health were enlightening and invaluable to my work on this book. Thanks to Clare Brigstocke and Wendy Jones for their many insights, Pattie Saluk for her reassuring words and keen medical eye, Hania Fedorowicz, for her editorial wisdom and acuity, Adam Mayers, Susan Mellan, Diane Mirabito, Gladys Mayers, John Goldup, Nancy Naples, Elana Rose and Dr. Howard Goodman for their helpful suggestions,

Paul Lessard and Laura Pratt for their help and availability at a moment's notice, and Raj Jalaladeen.

RESOURCES

Practitioners

Dr. Dana Colson, Doctor of Dental Surgery
1950 Yonge St, Toronto, Ontario M4S 1Z4
Phone 416-482-2133
Dr. Colson, integrates leading-edge science and technology with alternative wellness in her practice.

Dr. Fred Hui, M.D., integrative medicine
#201-421 Bloor St. E., Toronto, Ontario, M4W 3T1
Phone 416-920-4200
drhui@drhui.com
www.drhui.com
Dr. Hui is an integrative doctor who combines allopathic medicine, naturopathic medicine, traditional Chinese medicine, herbal interventions, and acupuncture in order to nourish the body and restore it to health through attention to the functioning of the kidneys, adrenal glands, and thyroid. His interventions can aid in re-balancing the body after chemotherapy and radiation.

Sat Dharam Kaur, Naturopathic doctor
Trillium Healing Arts Centre, 235 9th St. E., 2nd floor, Owen Sound, Ontario, N4K 1N8
Phone 519-372-9212
satdharamkaur@gmail.com
Sat Dharam Kaur developed and teaches The Healthy Breast Program in an effort to educate women in naturopathic ways to prevent and treat breast cancer. She published the excellent book The Complete Natural Medicine Guide to Breast Cancer.

Bernard Ma, Contact for Dr. Ma Hong Chau, Hong Kong
gatobma@gmail.com

Dr. Alex Mostovoy, Homeopath
3910 Bathurst St, Toronto, Ontario, M3H 5Z3
Phone 416-638-7555
www.drmostovoy.ca
Dr. Mostovoy is a homeopath and director of a medical thermography clinic. Thermography is a safe, radiation-free, painless process for screening for breast disease.

Dr. Abel Nasri, Naturopath, Homeopath, holistic health
Nasri Functional Medicine Clinic, 7611 Pine Valley Dr., Unit #7, Woodbridge, Ontario
Phone 905-266-0959
www.nasriclinic.ca
Dr. Nasri, who is also trained as a surgeon, is the director of the Alternative Holistic Health Services Clinic, where he specializes in treating cancers of all types at all stages.

Stanley Ngui, Acupuncturist
Ngui Integrative Medical Clinic and Qigong Studies, 165 East Beaver Creek Rd., Richmond Hill, Ontario, L4B 2N2
Phone 905-597-5007
nguistyleima@gmail.com
Stanley Ngui and his team specialize in treating patients who have or have had cancer.

Alvin Pettle, M.D., Gynecologist, integrative medicine
Ruth Pettle Wellness Centre, #207-3910 Bathurst St., North York, Ontario, M3H 5Z3
Phone 416-633-4011
info@drpettle.com
Dr. Pettle is an integrative medical doctor with a focus on bio-identical hormones. He is an expert in employing bio-identical hormones in the prevention and management of breast cancer.

Dr. Shaelendra Verma, Medical Oncologist,
The Ottawa Hospital, Room C2321, 501 Smyth Rd., Ottawa, Ontario K1H 8L6
Phone 613-737-7700 x70166
Dr. Verma supports the integration of naturopathic and complementary medicine within the traditional cancer care model, which is offered at the Ottawa Integrative Cancer Care treatment program.

Hua Allen Wang, Acupuncturist
Pain Relief Clinic, 425 Queen St. W., Unit #217, Toronto, Ontario, M5V 2A5
Phone 416-977-9853
Hua Allen Wang uses acupuncture alone or in combination with other alternative interventions to manage pain and immune system issues.

Compounding Pharmacies, Toronto

York Downs Pharmacy, 3910 Bathurst St., Toronto, Ontario, M3H 5Z3
Phone 416-633-2244
www.yorkdownsrx.com

Smith's Pharmacy, 3463 Yonge St., North York, Ontario, M4N 2N3
Phone 416-488-2600

Habers Compounding Pharmacy, 1584 Bathurst St., Toronto, Ontario, M5P 3H3
Phone 416-656-9830
info@haberspharmacy.com

Labs

Metametrix Clinical Lab, 3425 Corporate Way, Duluth, Georgia, 30096
Ion profile blood and urine testing.

Rocky Mountain Labs, 602 Park Point Dr. Suite #101, Golden, Colorado, 80401
Phone 1-800-776-5227
Urine testing to check ratios between two estrogen metabolytes, C2 and C16. These metabolytes, or products,are formed in the liver during the breakdown of estradiol and estrone. Determining their ratio, helps to understand how estrogen is being used in the body.

Meridian Valley Lab, 801 SW 16th St., Suite 126, Renton, WA, 98057
Phone 425-271-8689
Comprehensive hormone profiles.

Cancer Support Organizations, Toronto

Wellspring, 4 Charles St. E., Toronto, Ontario, M4Y 1T1
Phone 416-961-1928
Offers a range of programs and services which help with cancer recovery and restoring health and wellness for both patients and families.

Gilda's Club, 24 Cecil St., Toronto, Ontario, M5T 1N2
Phone 416-214-9898
info@gildasclubto.org
Offers various programs for those with a cancer diagnosis and their families to aid in dealing with diagnosis and recovery.

GLOSSARY

ACTH (adrenocorticotropic hormone): a hormone produced and secreted by the pituitary gland and often produced in response to biological stress. Its main effects are increased production and release of cortisol by the adrenal gland.

Adrenopause or adrenal fatigue: an imbalance of cortisol that causes hormone deficiencies.

Adjuvant treatment: treatment given after surgery that is administered to eradicate any cancer cells left behind.

Adriamycin: a chemotherapy drug, also known as Doxorubicin.

Antioxidants are substances that can prevent cell damage due to, for instance, free radicals.

Bioidentical hormones: natural hormones that women take to replace those that are depleted due to age or for other reasons. These hormones, when administered and monitored properly, do not increase breast density or increase breast cancer risk.

Biopsy: removing tissue in a suspicious area to determine if the cells are malignant.

Bisphenol A: is a chemical that acts as an endocrine disruptor. It is used in plastics in food and water containers, some metal products such as cans, some dental sealants and other products.

Cancer: most cases begin as a single cell or group of cells that mutate and multiply, creating abnormal cells that form a tumour.

Chemotherapy (chemo): targets cancer cells, (they are continually dividing), in order to stop the replication process. However chemo also damages normal cells.

Clean margins: when cancer cells do not extend to the outer edge of the tissue removed from the body.

Complementary medicine: involves combining treatments or substances that fall outside of conventional or mainstream treatments, such as acupuncture or nutritional supplementation, with mainstream medical interventions (e.g., employing acupuncture with chemo).

Contralateral prophylactic mastectomy (CPM): surgery on a woman who receives a diagnosis of breast cancer in one breast (unilateral breast cancer) and chose to have the other breast, which does not contain malignant tissue, removed as a preventive measure.

Cruciferous vegetables: include, for example, broccoli, cauliflower, brussel sprouts, and cabbage.

DCIS (ducal carcinoma in situ): a cancer that consists of abnormal cells; however, cell division is confined, it does not destroy local tissue, and it does not spread to distant sites.

Distal metastases: the often lethal spread of cancer from the primary site to other organs.

DNA (deoxyribonucleic acid): the molecular basis of heredity (genes). Cancer is caused by a chemical change or mutation in the DNA of one cell.

Ductal: arising from ducts within the breasts.

Early stage breast cancer: stages I and II.

Epstein Barr virus: a virus in the herpes family that causes mononucleosis.

Estrogen: a group of female hormones produced mainly in the ovaries and secondarily in the adrenal glands and fat cells.

Estrogen receptor positive cancer: a cancer in which the cancer cells receive signals from estrogen that could promote their growth.

Free radicals: are molecules generated by cells in the body. When excessive (they can be caused by, for instance, exposure to toxic chemicals, polluted air, alcohol, cigarette smoke), they damage genetic material and contribute to disease and aging.

Functional medicine: an approach to health that shifts the focus away from a conventional disease-centred approach to a patient-centred approach, viewing health as a systemic whole.

Gadolinium: a contrast dye often used in MRIs. It is known to be toxic, so it is chemically bonded in a particular way so that, when used with MRI, it will be eliminated from the body before it is released in the body's tissue. However, there is some evidence that it remains in the body.

Haemochromatosis: iron overload, an accumulation of iron in the body.

Herceptin is a drug that attaches itself to the HER2 receptors on the surface of the cancer cells and blocks them from receiving growth signals that stimulate uncontrolled growth. This medication can slow or stop breast cancer growth in those women whose breast cancer is driven by this process.

Herbal therapy: a method of medical treatment that involves mostly plants and plant extracts. In the early nineteenth century, scientists began making synthetic versions of plant compounds. As medical science began to flourish, herbal remedies were categorized as an alternative remedy.

Hormone therapy for breast cancer: a therapy targeting cells with receptors that attach to the hormones estrogen (ER-positive cancers) and/or progesterone (PR-positive cancers). Most types of hormone therapy for breast cancer either lower estrogen levels or stop estrogen from acting on breast cancer cells.

Immunoglobulin A (IgA): an antibody that plays a critical role in immune function in the mucous membranes. The IgA test measures the blood levels of immunoglobulin.

Immunoglobulins G (IgG) are antibodies that are produced by the body's immune system and are also closely linked to symptoms of food intolerance. Therefore this test, which helps detect antibodies to certain foods, can help determine which particular foods a person is reacting to.

In situ tumour: a small, completely localized, confined tumour.

Indole -3-carbinol: an anti-estrogenic substance found in cruciferous vegetables.

Infiltrating: invading the tissue immediately surrounding the tumour.

Integrative medicine: treatment that assumes that cancer requires a multifaceted approach and, therefore, combines mainstream with non-mainstream interventions (e.g., combining surgery and certain chemo treatments with for example nutrition, exercises, acupuncture, homeopathy).

Lumpectomy: surgical removal of a breast tumour and a small amount of surrounding tissue.

Malignant tumours: tumours that usually grow rapidly, destroying normal tissue and spreading to other parts of the body via the blood stream or by penetrating lymph channels and moving to lymph glands, and implanting themselves in other parts of the body, where they form what are called secondary tumours.

Mastectomy: a surgical procedure to remove the whole breast.

Melatonin: a hormone secreted in the pineal gland in the brain that regulates sleep and may have anti-cancer activity. It is also available as an artificial supplement.

Meta-analysis: the pooling of data from the existing research to distill all the data into one large study.

Metastatic: having spread elsewhere in the body.

MRI: a diagnostic tool that uses a magnetic field to produce images of organs and other internal structures. Unlike CT scans or X-rays, it does not use ionizing radiation that can cause DNA damage and cancer. However, the effects of exposure to MRI's magnetic fields are not known.

Myomin: an all-natural oral herbal formula is an aromatase inhibitor that helps with hormonal balance by blocking the aromatase enzyme. This reduces the production of estrogen. It also increases interferon and interleukin-2 production, which aid in stimulating natural killer cells and enhancing the body's ability to fight tumour cells.

Naturopathy: a medical system based on helping the body to heal itself using natural substances and non-invasive techniques.

Node negative: no evidence of cancer in lymph nodes.

PCB (polychlorinated biphenyl): an organic chlorine compound known to be a neurotoxin and to have endocrine-disruption properties.

PET (positron emission tomography) scan: an image that uses a radioactive drug to determine how tissues and organs are functioning.

Screening mammogram: a mammogram done on a woman with no palpable lump and no obvious signs of breast cancer, often done at regular intervals.

Stage: an indication of the size of the cancer and how far it has spread.

Stage I: a small (2 centimetres or less) cancerous breast tumour with no cancer in lymph nodes.

Stage II: a small tumour with limited cancer found in lymph nodes, or a tumour over 2 centimetres in size with no cancer in lymph nodes.

Tamoxifen: an estrogen-blocking drug.

SELECTED BIBLIOGRAPHY

Agus, David. *The End of Illness.* New York: Free Press, Simon and Schuster, 2011

Austin, Steve and Hitchcock, Cathy. *What You Should Know (But May Not Be Told) About Prevention, Diagnosis, and Treatment.* California: Prima Publishing, 1994

Brody, Theodore. *Alkalize or Die.* North Carolina: Holographic Health Press, 1991

Epstein, Samuel S. *Cancer Gate.* New York: Baywood Publishing Company, 2005

Kaur, Sat Dharam, *The Complete Natural Medicine Guide to Breast Cancer*, Toronto: Robert Rose, 2003

Krop, Joseph. *Healing the Planet One Patient at a Time: A Primer in Environmental Medicine.* Alton, Ontario: Kos Publishing, 2002

Lee, John R. et al, *What Your Doctor Might Not Tell You About Breast Cancer. How Hormone Balance Can Help Save your Life.* New York: Warner books, 2002

Mukherjee, Siddhartha. *The Emperor of All Maladies.* New York: Scribner, 2010

Plant, Jane. *Your life in Your Hands: Understand, Prevent and Overcome Breast Cancer and Ovarian Cancer*. UK: Ebury Publishing, 2007

Robbins, John. *Diet For a New America. How Your Food Choices Affect Your Health, Happiness, and the Future of Life on Earth*. Novato, California: New World Library, 2012

Servan-Schreiber, David. *Anticancer: A New Way of Life*. New York: Penguin, 2008.

Steingraber, Sandra. *Living Downstream: An Ecologist Looks at Cancer and the Environment*.Reading, Mass. Addison-Wesley Publishing, 1997

Teitelbaum, Jacob. *From Fatigued to Fantastic*. London, England: Penguin, 2007.

INDEX

biophysical 49, 109

biopsy/biopsies 3, 13, 39, 40, 55, 58, 88, 109

Bisphenol A 99, 102, 103

biteplates 102

bladder 79, 80

bleeding 93

blood 5, 10, 12, 17, 25, 27-29, 31, 40, 56, 58, 60, 62, 63, 75, 92, 95, 99-102, 106, 107, 111, 127, 137, 142

blood clots 31

bone 5, 31, 45, 62, 73, 94, 99-102, 104, 112, 135, 136

bones 62, 64, 132, 141

boost immune system 60, 144

botanicals 73

bowel(s) 33, 56, 92, 93

BPA 102, 103

brain 43, 55, 62, 67, 68, 81, 93

brassica 26

breakthrough, in medical treatment 80
    targeting bad genes 85

breast 1, 3, 4, 6-10, 12-15, 21, 23-43, 45-51, 53, 55, 56, 58, 59, 61, 62, 64, 66-68, 71, 73, 77-79, 81, 82, 85-89, 100, 103, 104, 106-111, 115-138, 141, 143, 144, 146, 147

breasts 39, 40, 51, 55, 67, 103, 109, 115, 129, 130, 143

breathing, mercury 93, 131

British 13, 33, 70, 88, 119, 121, 122, 129

broccoli 26, 44, 63, 68

bromocriptine 70, 71

Brusch, Charles 11

burdock 11

C

cadmium 103

cancer(s) 1, 3-19, 21, 23-56, 57, 58, 59, 60, 61-74, 77-91, 93, 94, 102-112, 115-141, 143, 144, 146-149

oral health and intestinal health 93
contaminants, in environment 96
contraindications 45, 69, 143
contralateral 129-131
controversial, Dr. Di Bella 70
    mammography screening 118
Copenhagen 121
coronary 131
cortisol 36, 38, 41-43, 46, 108, 142
C-reactive protein 29, 107, 144
cream, DHEA 43
    progesterone 46
estriol 68, 108, 109, 142
crown, dental 98, 102, 142
cruciferous vegetables 27, 44, 68
CT scan (computerized tomography) 55
cumulative, effects of radiation 55
    mammography screening 124
curative, homeopathy 10
factors 90
curcumin 27, 28, 106
cure, cancer 10, 11, 15, 48, 50, 56, 63, 65, 66, 70, 74, 77, 78,
    80, 81, 82, 83, 84, 85, 88, 118, 120, 133, 134, 144, 146, 147,
    148, 149
cycle(s), menstrual 67, 86
cyclophosphamide 70, 71
cysteine 97
cystic 40

D

dairy 13, 63, 94
    dairy-free 63, 141
damage 65

F

food(s) 12, 13, 15, 17, 18, 26, 27, 33, 45, 63, 68, 72, 92, 94, 96, 105, 110, 126
foreign, bodies 12
     implants 102
foxglove, purple 84
fracture, teeth 102
fruit(s) 32, 44
functioning 18, 29, 59, 69
     immune 60, 64, 106, 110
     thyroid, adrenal, kidney 75, 76, 110
fungal 25, 29, 30, 75
fungi 93

G
gadolinium 127
gamma, delta cells 11
gastrointestinal 79, 92
gene(s) 30, 32, 36, 50, 80, 85, 124, 134
     therapy 80, 85
     HER2 116
     test 135
genesis 80, 81
genetic(s) 25, 32, 36, 39, 41, 42, 49, 58, 60, 79, 80, 81, 85, 105, 107, 117, 123, 125, 136, 141, 147
genitourinary, cancer 79
Germany, chronomodulated chemo 60
germinate, cancer 69
Gladwell, Malcolm 123, 124
gland(s) 11, 42, 51, 67, 68, 75, 107-109
glucose 33, 44, 93
glutathione 60, 97, 107
gluten-free 63
glycemic 27
grade 138 nuclear 115
     differentiation 116

K

kefir 141
kelp 26, 27, 107
kidney(s) 33, 76, 93, 109
    killer cells 12, 60, 80, 143
Krop, Joseph 12
Kundalini 13

L

lactic acid 33
laser 100
late-stage cancers 57
leakage, dental amalgam 96
leaky gut 94, 97
lesions 122
    and tumour markers 59, 110
        cellular abnormalities and benign lesions 120, 121, 125, 125
leukemia 30, 74, 117
lipoic acid 59,60, 107
liver 15, 16, 18, 24, 28, 29, 33, 38, 42-44, 60-62, 74, 75, 93,
    106, 142
lobular 50, 51
low-dose chemo 57, 60, 70
    toxins 94
low-grade, infection 28, 100
    prostate cancer 83,
lump 12, 37, 40, 54, 58, 67, 69, 118, 144
lumpectomy 59, 78, 79, 82, 110, 111, 122, 128, 129, 133
lung(s) 13, 26, 55, 62, 66, 81, 92, 93, 95, 111, 117, 133, 134, 142
lymph nodes 6, 37, 41, 42, 88
lymphatic(s) 33, 50, 88
lymphedema 88
lymphocytes 75
lymphomas(s) 33, 71, 74

M

N

O

P

positive, estrogen, progesterone, HER2 4, 31, 38, 41, 42, 45, 46,
116, 122, 135, 136
biopsies 55
post-diagnosis, survival after radiation 133, 140
posttreatment, acupuncture 142
predictive, thermography 55
cancer biology 123
oncotype 135
predisposition 41, 141
genetic and mammography 125
pregnancy 45 breast cancer protection 87
premenopausal 124, 136
premenstrual syndrome, and excessive estrogen 67, 109
preventative, bio-identical hormones 35, 68, 69, 109
exercise 19, 33, 38, 44, 52, 87, 91, 107, 108, 112, 148
prevention, cancer 12, 21, 106
melatonin 69, 80, 106, 115
mammograph 143
primary 51
treatment 88
surgery 111
treatment 136
probiotics 28, 106, 141
progesterone 4, 9, 10, 31, 45, 46, 61, 66, 67, 87, 107-109,
116, 135
progestin 47
prognosis, stages 54, 56, 116
sentinel node biopsy 88
tumour size 117, 123
alternative remedies 141
propolis 6
prostate 58, 66, 79, 80, 83, 85
protocol 9, 24, 27, 34, 48, 59, 61, 62, 70, 71, 75, 97, 110, 112,
117, 118,134, 146, 148
PSA 58, 83

pseudo-pregnancy 87

pulse 17, 18

Q

quinoa 44

R

radiation 4, 6, 8, 9, 12-14, 18, 23, 25, 26, 37, 41, 42, 52, 54-56, 59, 60, 74, 77-79, 81-85, 88, 107-110, 115, 118, 122, 124, 125, 127, 128, 131-133, 138-141, 143-145

radical, mastectomies 28, 77, 78, 129

radioactive, molecules 26, 107

raw food 13, 94

receptors, estriol 45

    progesterone-positive 46

    estrogen positive 31, 44, 61, 68, 103

recover(ies) 18, 24, 52, 72, 74,75, 109

recurrence(s) 6, 13, 16, 19, 25, 27, 28, 30-34, 38, 52, 53, 64, 66, 68, 69, 74, 82, 87, 89, 90, 107, 111, 128, 131, 132, 136, 139-141

    prevention 13, 28, 29, 67, 109, 133

reflexology 61

regressed, some invasive breast cancers 123

reiki 61, 90

Reishi 27

relapse 88, 89, 134

remission 16, 45, 59

resection 15

residues, animal hormones 68

    fish 94

resveratrol 11

retinoids 70, 71

reverse, chemo/radiation damage 23, 52

    breast cancer 26, 33, 42, 50, 64, 104

Richards, Gordon 78

T

transvaginal 142

tubules, dentin 99

tumour(s) 9, 12, 16, 18, 25, 29, 30, 31, 33, 40, 43, 50, 51, 53, 54, 58, 61, 89, 110, 115, 123-126, 133, 134, 143

   markers 59, 60, 62, 70, 81, 82, 85, 88, 89, 107, 108, 110, 115-118, 122

   size 123-126, 133, 134, 138, 141, 143, 146

turmeric 26, 27, 126, 142

U

Ukrain 72

ultrasound 3, 10, 16, 28, 39, 40, 45, 55, 56, 58, 108, 118, 144

under-oxygenated, hypoxic 42

urination , frequent 75

urine tests 27-29, 43, 46, 70, 106

uterine cancer 31, 67

V

vagina(l) 43, 46, 89, 108, 142

vaginally, estriol 44, 45

vegan 32, 75

vegetarian 41, 44

Verma, Shailendra 86, 111

virus 17, 30, 49, 66, 73-75

virus-based cancers 66

vitamin, C 26, 27, 33, 60, 71, 97, 107, 109, 141

   D 29, 107, 109, 141

   K2 94, 142

   Poly MVA 57

Vitex 61

W

Wachter, Robert 147

water, intake 10, 38, 44, 108

   nightguard 102

ABOUT THE AUTHOR

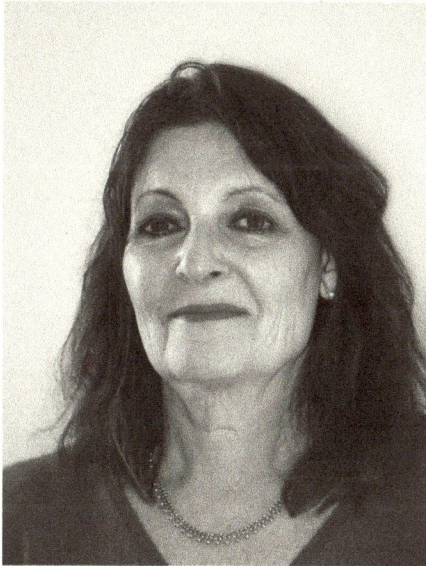

Aviva Mayers, MSW., is a psychoanalyst and has worked as a clinical social worker in hospitals in several countries. She lived and worked in Canada, the U.K., the U.S. and Norway where she pursued post graduate studies at the Norwegian University of Science and Technology, while also teaching and working in private practice. She now lives in Toronto where she treats individuals and couples in her private practice. Her experience with breast cancer has taught her that if we take responsibility for our own health by informing ourselves and employing interventions that make sense to us, we can improve our health and transform our lives.

Printed in May 2021
by Rotomail Italia S.p.A., Vignate (MI) - Italy